Own Your Fertility

Own Your Fertility

From Egg Freezing to Surrogacy, How to Take Charge of Your Body and Your Future

Jaime Knopman, MD

with Rebecca Raphael

Countryman Press

An Imprint of W. W. Norton & Company
Independent Publishers Since 1923

OWN YOUR FERTILITY is a general information resource about fertility preservation. It is not a substitute for individual medical diagnosis or treatment. The names and potentially identifying characteristics of patients mentioned in this book have been changed. Any URLs displayed in this book link or refer to websites that existed as of press time. The publisher is not responsible for, and should not be deemed to endorse or recommend, any resource referred to, any website other than its own, or any app or content that it did not create. The authors, also, are not responsible for any third-party material.

For information about permission to reproduce selections from this book, write to Permissions, Countryman Press, 500 Fifth Avenue, New York, NY 10110

For information about special discounts for bulk purchases, please contact W. W. Norton Special Sales at specialsales@wwnorton.com or 800-233-4830

Manufacturing by Lakeside Book Company
Production manager: Devon Zahn

Countryman Press
www.countrymanpress.com

An imprint of W. W. Norton & Company, Inc.
500 Fifth Avenue, New York, NY 10110
www.wwnorton.com

Authorized EU representative: EAS, Mustamäe tee 50, 10621 Tallinn, Estonia

978-1-324-11148-1

10 9 8 7 6 5 4 3 2 1

To the triangle, Charley and Blake.
I life you.

Contents

Author's Note

I AM WRITING THIS BOOK as a white, cisgender, heterosexual, college-educated woman and as a physician who has devoted my career to providing reproductive care to all women. While this book draws primarily on my decades of medical training and expertise providing counseling and treatment to individuals and couples, it also incorporates my opinions based on my lived experiences, including as a parent. The practice of medicine is my professional calling, but being a parent is the ultimate joy and gift of my life—so I want that deeply for my patients, too, if that is what they desire. Every single day, raising my two daughters reinforces my boundless commitment to fertility education and my passion to provide all people the support they need to create a family of their own in whatever way is right for them.

While healthcare may not be equitable, all people are capable of learning about their bodies so that they can make informed choices based on their reproductive potential and the factors that may impact it. Choosing parenthood is a personal decision that is not right for everyone. Having biological children (or any children) is not a prerequisite for living a whole, meaningful life. I am advocating for people to make whatever choices suit them from a place of knowledge, empowerment, and proactivity, particularly as the options available in the field of fertility have transformed in recent years and will continue to evolve.

Own Your Fertility is not meant to be used in lieu of individualized medical care, serve as a medical textbook, or provide answers to specific medical questions. Decisions on treatment should always be discussed with your physician or medical team, hopefully as part of what I like to think of as a sacred dialogue. My objective is to help you supplement such conversations and care, not replace them.

I support a diverse patient population and am accepting of all individuals who desire to partner with me throughout any part of their fertility journey. In this book, I will use the terms *woman, women,* or *female* to refer to people with one or more ovaries; however, I recognize that not everyone with such internal reproductive organs identifies as a woman or a female. In fact, I recently froze the eggs of a transgender man who kept his ovaries and uterus in order to be able to carry and subsequently deliver a child—which he did. I am choosing not to use gender-neutral language because the majority of my patients identify as female and the majority of patients globally who get pregnant are women. I trained as an obstetrician and gynecologist, am board certified in reproductive endocrinology and infertility, and have continued to primarily focus on the reproductive care of women. I do see male patients who struggle with infertility, but fertility services, especially in the realm of preservation, are more frequently accessed by females.

All the patient anecdotes I share are real, but the names and some identifying features have been changed.

Introduction:
The Fertility Unfair-y Tale

FERTILITY IS NOT FAIR TO WOMEN. Far from it. Women are born with all the eggs we will ever have, and we start losing them before we are even out of the womb. While most men produce millions of new sperm every day, women can never make new eggs, and the ones we do have start declining precipitously in both quantity and quality in our early 30s. That slope of decline grows even steeper quite quickly. Ninety percent of a woman's eggs are gone by age 30, making it increasingly difficult to become pregnant around the same time that many women are focused on finding a life partner, building their career, or, as I see most commonly in my medical practice, both. Women sure got the short end of the fertility stick.

We've known how unfair fertility is for a long time, and women have heard the unavoidable ticking of their biological clocks all the while. And didn't we all learn in elementary school that life isn't fair? But when something isn't fair, I believe in taking action—smart, strategic, measured action. When it comes to our fertility, we are not powerless, especially nowadays. As I tell my patients, stop lamenting the biological status quo or wallowing in self-pity and do something! We have agency. That ticking biological clock doesn't need to feel like a time bomb. Now more than ever, it is neither a clock without a "snooze" button nor an explosive.

Science has advanced, the world we live in has transformed, and the choices we make can now change, too. Thanks to Assisted Reproductive

Technology (ART), which is the umbrella term for any procedure in which eggs or embryos are manipulated outside of the body, we are able to tackle what I consider one of the last bastions of feminism: providing women real choices and increasing access to reproductive freedom. By freezing reproductive tissue like eggs or considering other treatments for fertility preservation, women can build their careers, find partners, explore their passions, get pregnant, and build families on their own timetable—aging eggs be damned. As a physician in one of the country's top fertility practices, I help women do exactly this.

If you asked me five years ago what kind of doctor I was, I would have told you I was a reproductive endocrinologist specializing in *infertility*. Most of my patients were couples who had been trying to get pregnant, to no avail; it was my job to help them figure out why it wasn't happening and what we could do about it. I also treated single women, usually in their late 30s or early 40s, who feared they had run out of time to find a partner with whom to build a family, so they were opting to try for parenthood with donor sperm. Now I consider myself a *fertility* specialist. In some circles, particularly in New York City, I've become known as the Queen of Egg Freezing. Now that science has possibilities for women who may want to preserve their fertility, I can help patients achieve their dream of becoming a parent without an unyielding biological clock running the show. This shift is profound, as everything about the way we can make babies has changed.

Nearly 70 percent of the patients I saw last year, most in their late 20s or early 30s, were there for fertility preservation as opposed to treating infertility. Rather than coming to my office consumed by anguish and fear, many of my patients are boldly planning for their future before their deteriorating eggs narrow down their options for them. No desperation, only strategic decision-making and empowerment. I treat single women who undergo egg freezing so they can take their time looking for a partner with whom to build a family without sacrificing egg quality. I support same-sex couples who will need IVF when they decide to start a family, and I work with heterosexual couples who may want flexibility with their timetable for having kids. I also treat patients who don't know if they will want to have kids one day, but they are choosing to exercise the reproductive options that are available so they may have the possibility of genetic parenthood in years to come. Also, whereas my practice used to cater primarily to one-percenters who could afford expensive procedures or upper-middle-class patients who were spending every last dime they had saved, increasingly my patients have employers that foot the bill.

This seismic shift is playing out nationally and globally as well. In just the three years between 2019 and 2022, in the midst of the COVID-19 pandemic, the number of ART procedures across the country increased 30 percent. That in itself is a huge jump in a short time span, but what's even more astounding to me is that more than one-third of those cycles were egg or embryo freezing cycles, in which all of the eggs or embryos were cryopreserved for future use. I can't tell you why each one of those people chose to freeze eggs or embryos, but I can say with certainty that ART for purposes of fertility preservation, as opposed to for infertility treatment, has taken off. Similar trends have played out across the globe, including the United Kingdom, Spain, Australia, New Zealand, Japan, Ireland, and France. Post-pandemic, of the more than 400,000 IVF cycles performed in 2022 throughout the United States, approximately 40 percent were frozen and intended for future use. In other words, the number of overall IVF procedures and the percentage that are for fertility preservation are continuing to grow substantially. As I've seen in my own practice, ART has become not just more accessible but also more affordable as the number of employers offering expansive fertility benefits has expanded significantly in all sectors.

The rapidly and drastically changing fertility landscape is about so much more than how, when, and with whom we may try to become a parent. When women have the ability to give their biological clock a time-out with fertility preservation, they can make choices about their education, career, life partner, or anything else that fulfills them without paying the price of an increased risk of infertility. As the average age of a person giving birth for the first time rises, as it has been consistently since the 1970s, more women are staying in the workforce and achieving financial independence. According to US Census studies, delaying childbirth by five years results in an average salary increase of $16,000. From my vantage as a working mom, that's a win—all the more so when women can postpone parenthood hopefully without compromising egg quality.

As the Director of Fertility Preservation in the United States and Canada for the Colorado Center for Reproductive Medicine (CCRM), a pioneer in fertility science, research, and treatment, I am privileged to both watch the field advance and help women, men, and couples pursue the right option for them. When I guide someone grieving the loss of fertility to an alternate path to parenthood, I am moved to tears of joy time and time again. When extracting and freezing eggs allows women to press pause so they can date without being consumed by fear that time is running out, or prioritize other ambitions before starting a family, it is inspiring. When I work with same-sex couples to create the family of their dreams, I marvel at how far both science and society have come.

Fertility is not a birthright (pun intended). You may not get a happily ever after with the love of your life, and even if you do, getting pregnant can be hard. Not everyone wants children or knows if they may possibly want children one day. But if you want to keep that door open, or if you have a loved one for whom you value reproductive options, you must be informed and intentional. Your ovaries will not wait for you, but you can take ownership of your reproduction. (Psst! The earlier the better.)

So who is *Own Your Fertility* intended for? Just about everyone: Those who want children now, or maybe one day, or aren't sure if they ever will; those who have struggled to get pregnant or have never even tried; those who trust in the power of ART or are skeptical; those who have comprehensive medical benefits or limited resources; those who are straight, gay, or any other sexual orientation; those who are single, in a relationship, or have varied definitions of what a family means; those who "want it all" or who think that's an unrealistic ideal; those who have eggs, sperm, or neither. No matter your circumstances or goals, I hope to inspire you to take charge of your reproductive journey armed with scientific data, my perspectives, others' experiences, and hard-earned takeaways.

I haven't worn my white lab coat in years because it felt like a hierarchical barrier between my patients and me. I prefer to talk to them like they are my friends or younger sisters, with directness, authenticity, and respect—

just as I will do with you. I ask my patients to call me by my first name because I think of myself as a partner, not just an expert. It is my life's work to contribute to the revolution that is catalyzing people, especially women, to become thoughtful and proactive about their reproduction. I am honored to also partner with you in the pages that follow to help you make informed, authentic, courageous, and empowering decisions. You really *can* own your fertility, starting now and for many years to come.

PART 1

PRESERVING YOUR FERTILITY

CHAPTER 1

Why You Need a Fertility Plan

I LOVE A GOOD PLAN. There's nothing in my life I don't plan (or at least try to). From my marathon training schedule to a monthly calendar of what's for dinner for my family, I have all kinds of systems because I can't function without them. I loathe wasted time, value measurable outcomes, and thrive sticking to the programs I craft. I have always been this way. Some of my plans have worked out exceptionally well, but some pretty big ones have exploded in my face. So why should you listen to me about the importance of having a plan, which is what this chapter is all about, when some of mine have blown up in smoke and left me in the fetal position, ugly crying? Just stay with me.

I knew I wanted to be a doctor after reading a book in second grade about Elizabeth Blackwell, the first female physician in the United States. I was fascinated by science, particularly biology, liked solving problems, and wanted to help people. I had always been a very diligent student who followed the rules, earned accolades, set goals, and then executed my plans to reach them. Thanks to incredibly hard work, supportive parents, federal loans, a dose of luck—and all my plans—as soon as I decided that medicine was the field for me, I earned my undergraduate degree, an MD, and a white coat with my name embroidered on it. I developed a passion for women's health, particularly for reproductive endocrinology (all things hormones), which had me feeling like I was conducting a beautiful orchestra, with the brain, ovaries, uterus, and hormones each playing a powerful role.

Perhaps like you, I wanted to get married and have kids. That plan started to take shape when I met another first-year med student on the very first day of our program. We quickly fell in love, matched for our respective residencies in top programs in the same city, and then got married when I was 27. After we completed our fellowships, won coveted medical awards, and got the jobs we each wanted in New York City, we had two daughters. When I became a mom, I felt a kind of love I had never known before. My magical experience of parenthood was a gift I wanted to share with others, provided that's what they wanted for themselves. I continued to deliver babies, remove uteri, extract eggs, and transfer embryos with an intensified desire to help others achieve their family goals. From being married to a surgeon to pumping breast milk in between surgeries and racing home to read the girls our favorite book, *I Love You Forever*, I felt like I was living a *Grey's Anatomy* cliché. By the time I was 36, I had essentially checked all my boxes. My plans were right on track.

My naive vision of happily ever after took a detour. My tried-and-true linear plans didn't account for my husband unexpectedly asking for a divorce. We were supposed to make it to our 50th wedding anniversary and beyond, just like my parents had. That was the plan! No matter how darn cute our holiday card had been for years, my girls would never grow up with a picture-perfect family. I was 39, my girls were six and three, and my plans were shattered. So was I. Even once my ex-husband had moved out of our apartment and I hadn't worn my wedding band in months, I remember staring at my Facebook profile, petrified to press the key that would change my status from Married to Single. In my narrow mind, it was as if that one keystroke was announcing to the world I had gone off course, that I hadn't achieved all I had set out to accomplish, that my seemingly perfect life was actually in shambles. I pitied myself, I wondered if others pitied me, and I was ashamed. Despite becoming a board-certified doctor who helped people every day, my formula of over-planning, overstudying, and overtraining seemed useless in a world that could be cruelly unpredictable. Some things in life were simply out of my control. Imagine that.

Soon after our split, just when I was getting my sea legs as a divorced working mom of two little girls in third grade and kindergarten, I discovered a lump in my left breast. It turned out to be malignant cancer, and I had a double mastectomy after my 41st birthday. It was the hardest chapter of my life. Not for one minute did I stop feeling grateful that I had found the lump, had access to treatment, and was expected to make a full recovery, but I was petrified and felt broken. How had my life veered so far off track from all I had brazenly strategized? My plans had failed me. I had failed me. This was not how it was supposed to be.

I would ultimately discover that the path to the life I wanted hadn't disappeared overnight; I just needed to be comfortable with an unexpected (and sometimes painful) turn or two. My life may have taken a couple of detours—divorce and cancer—but my plans still led me to where I am now. Day in and day out, I get to help others carve out a path to parenthood or lay the foundation for that possibility in the future. I am remarried to my forever life partner, cancer-free, and have a beautiful blended family in a loving, chaotic home. My dreams of making it to my 50th anniversary like my parents may not turn out as I had hoped, but my husband and I can have a blowout party for our 25th. I still love plans.

My patients often ask if I struggled with fertility. I did not. I was also fortunate to have had my kids before my breast cancer diagnosis and subsequent treatment, which could have impacted my fertility. My empathy and fervor to support other women comes from a different place than personal experience with infertility. When my marriage and my health went downhill, I was compelled to reexamine my people-pleasing, box-checking, perfection-driven life strategies. By sitting in my own pain and growing from it, I learned that the deviations from my strategically orchestrated plans were not failure. Quite the contrary. I love what I do as a physician, and the winding roads I was forced to take in life make me even better at it. I understand grief and heartache in a profound way that has me connect intimately with my patients, many of whom are struggling to accept circumstances they never expected nor wanted. When I work with people who are lost in a sea of hopelessness, I understand how paralyzing unforeseen circumstances can be.

As I embrace midlife, I am able to make sense of how my hardships have given me a renewed sense of purpose to help others. I am still an optimist. I still believe everything happens for a reason, and I know that after every rainstorm there is a rainbow—if you stick around long enough. I have a keen sense of gratitude, particularly for having my kids before the demise of my marriage. Being their mom, whether I'm married, divorced, or remarried, is the biggest blessing of my lifetime. I now appreciate that there is not one path forward in any aspect of life, including marriage, fertility, parenting, and beyond. I still very much believe in having a plan, even though life is unpredictable. We should not go into any chapter of our life blind, and certainly not when it comes to reproduction.

The Other Plan B

I cannot count the number of women who have come up to me in the gym locker room asking, "You're the fertility doctor, right? I'm 37. Should I freeze my eggs?" I'm standing there half naked, drenched in sweat, being asked to dispense advice to women who may have spent more time planning their workout regimen than they did thinking about how or when they might consider maximizing their precious and fading fertility. I have seen thousands of women who did almost everything according to plan, from top-tier educations to six-figure jobs, and just assumed building a family would fall into place. They end up in my office lamenting lost time, lost love, and essentially, lost eggs. They ask, "Why me? What did I do wrong while everyone else found a spouse and became a mom? Why was I the one who got left behind? What should I have done differently?"

My answer, delivered not with a wagging finger but with compassion, is usually something like this: "First of all, you are not alone. Not everyone else got a fairytale ending while you got left behind. I promise you that. Secondly, amid all your plans, did you have one for fertility? All women need a fertility plan so their biology does not dictate the future. I'm sorry you were not told that sooner. It is not fair, but let's do what we can to change that now."

In a 2022 interview with *Allure* magazine, Jennifer Aniston said,

"I would've given anything if someone had said to me: 'Freeze your eggs. Do yourself a favor.' You just don't think it. So here I am today. The ship has sailed." But the ship has not sailed for everyone. So here I am to say it to you: Women, who are born with all the eggs they will ever have and lose them faster than they may want, need to know the basic facts about their bodies and the options for exerting some control over reproductive choices. Getting educated about the opportunities to defy your biology and put your body in the best possible position to support long-term goals can provide freedom, empowerment, and life-changing options.

We have fire drills and school shooter drills to prepare for circumstances we hope will never happen. We are taught about the importance of a financial plan because winging it when the time comes to pay for college or to retire is shortsighted. We wear seat belts when we get in a car and helmets when we ride a bicycle to help shield us in unforeseen circumstances. We also have all kinds of insurance offerings like disability, auto, fire, pet, flood, or homeowners, to provide a safety net for scenarios that may or may not come to pass. It is possible your flood insurance will be useless depending on the cause, and a spike in your car insurance premium after an accident may cost more than just paying out of pocket. But insurance still typically gives us peace of mind and can protect us, whether financially or otherwise. Now, thanks to modern medicine and reproductive technologies, I am suggesting that women consider an insurance policy of sorts when it comes to reproduction, a safety net that entails having a fertility plan.

Nothing in life is without risk or failure. People get pregnant while using condoms or on the pill, but I sure as hell still want my daughters to use contraception when they become sexually active. ART is about choice, not control. I am a doer. I don't believe in sitting back passively, no matter what life throws at me. I come at this from a place of not just medical expertise but a bias toward proactivity. You want to run faster? Go train. Aiming to do better on an exam? Study harder. Goal is to lose weight? Prioritize nutrition and exercise. And if you want to have the option of extending your fertility, then I recommend making smart choices today to maximize your chance of success in the future.

I hope your life goes according to plan, whether you have one or many. But in case it doesn't, I suggest having what I call the "Other Plan B." The regular Plan B is a type of emergency contraception also known as the morning-after pill. The Other Plan B I'm talking about applies to the other end of the reproductive spectrum: treatments like egg freezing and IVF that can help people build families with a push from modern medicine. Such a plan starts with getting informed about your body and the choices for how and when to procreate.

Like many aspects of women's health that have gotten shortchanged for decades, education about reproduction and the most recent advancements in the field have not been highlighted. Reproductive medicine is a field that is rife with bioethical, religious, moral, and political considerations. We don't yet know what quandaries may await as technology and medicine advance at lightning speed. But potential objections or concerns about those options should not deter us from educating people about their very existence. There are choices you may never want to utilize. Or you may make plans to take advantage of them if needed and never choose to implement them. Or your Other Plan B may become key to fulfilling a dream of parenthood. None of us knows what the future holds, but we do know that infertility is inevitable as we age. The advent of treatments for fertility preservation can liberate you to make decisions without the previously inescapable ticking of a clock guiding—or misguiding—you.

Birth Control vs. Controlling Birth

For most people, the first part of making their fertility plan (probably without even realizing that's what they're doing) is taking precautions to *not* get pregnant. Such a plan may involve choosing abstinence or using birth control options ranging from condoms, the pill, IUDs, vaginal rings, patches, or a combination thereof. To me, birth control—especially the pill, with its 99 percent effectiveness when used correctly—is science's greatest gift to women. That high likelihood of not getting pregnant, enabled by just popping a pill, has given us the freedom to have sex, build careers, focus on our education, or make any other life choice without unwanted pregnancy as a factor to consider.

Avoiding getting pregnant is one aspect of birth control, and an important one at that. But I also think of birth control through the lens of controlling our ability to have a baby. We need to think about and plan for the possibility of getting pregnant just as much—if not more—than we think about and plan for how *not* to get pregnant. Getting pregnant doesn't happen as easily as we think it might, especially when we choose to try at a later age than previous generations. Once a woman is in her 20s, I recommend that annual visits to a healthcare provider—whether it's a general practitioner, OB-GYN, or fertility specialist—include conversations about a fertility plan.

Most of the women I see for fertility preservation consultations are pretty sure they will want to have children one day, but that is not always the case. Sometimes my patients' parents come in with their grown children in hopes that grandparenthood remains a possibility for them, so they are the ones steering the ship (and footing the bill). I also see plenty of women who have not given much thought to parenthood, but they want to keep their options open while they have other priorities for the next decade, perhaps work or travel. Many couples come into my office as they begin to think about getting engaged, married, or starting their family planning. Quite often that's when and where they discover that they aren't on the same page because they never took the time to get real about some of the tough questions we all need to be asking.

In all of my consultations, these are some of the questions I ask as a starting point for anyone beginning to create a fertility plan:

» How old are you?
» Do you get regular periods? How many days are between your periods and for how long do you bleed? Are your periods painful?
» Have you ever required surgery on your uterus, your ovaries, or your cervix?
» Are you sexually active with men, women, or both?
» Do you currently use birth control? If yes, what kind? Have you previously been on another type of birth control?
» Have you ever tried to get pregnant? Have you ever been pregnant?

» If you have been pregnant, did it end in a delivery, a miscarriage, or a termination?

» Do you know if you want to have children one day? Do you want to have biological children? If you're not sure, would you like to keep that option available to you?

» If you do hope to have children, how many might you want to try to have?

» Do you have an ideal timeline for when you might want to become a parent?

» Do you have a partner? If yes, is this the partner with whom you may want to have children? Are you and your partner on the same page about having a family together and a possible timeline?

» If you don't have a partner, are you hoping to find one before considering parenthood? Are you open to single parenthood?

» Is there anything that you are aware of that might prevent you from carrying a pregnancy?

» Have you had any significant medical problems or a family history of serious illness like cancer?

» Might you be a carrier of a dominant condition such as BRCA? Have you done any genetic testing to know if you are a carrier for any recessive conditions?

» Has anyone in your family experienced infertility, early menopause, or recurrent miscarriage?

» Are you or your partner an only child? Do you know if that was by choice?

» If you have a partner, have they done any genetic testing? Do you know the results?

» If you have a partner, have they had any significant medical problems or a family history of serious illness?

» If you have a partner, have they ever achieved a pregnancy?

» If you have a male partner, has he ever had a semen analysis? Do you know the results?

» Do you hope to use your own eggs to conceive?

» Do you want to carry a pregnancy?

» Do you have any fears surrounding conception and parenthood in general?

» If you are hesitant about trying to get pregnant, what may be holding you back?

» Do you work at a company that provides fertility benefits? If yes, what do they entail and when do they expire? Might you leave your job in the near or distant future, whether electively or not by your own choice?

» Where do you live, and do you have any plans to move?

» What do you hope your future looks like, whether you have big-picture dreams or specific goals? Do you have a vision of success or, conversely, of failure?

When I meet a new patient or couple, I go from "Nice to meet you" to some version of "What fears keep you up at night?" within the span of an hour. If I am going to help my patients come up with a short- or long-term plan that is right for them, we've got to be honest with each other and ourselves. My goal is not to be offensive or intrusive, but to make sure patients are thoughtful about their goals, have the opportunity to achieve them, and keep me abreast of changes in circumstances, hopes, and obstacles.

The same goes for you. You've got to start somewhere, so take the time to start thinking about these questions based on your present-day circumstances and future hopes. I suggest you discuss your answers with your physician so you can begin to formulate a fertility plan that is right for you. Your answers may change from year to year. In fact, I hope they do, because that is all part of the journey. Life is not a straight line and detours are inevitable, so the plans you make by the end of this book could become nothing more than pivot points in the years to come. That's why many of my patients who choose not to pursue fertility treatment right away come back to me, so we can reassess how their life has changed, and we can be sure they are still positioned to possibly achieve what they want down the road. Not all doctors have been trained to think along these lines, so if your medical professional does not initiate such a conversation, you can and should. Again, these are conversations to be having annually starting in your 20s, not as a one-off consultation.

Changing World, Changing Choices

As a physician in a national practice with offices in 26 cities throughout the United States and Canada, I am privy to not just *how* fertility treatment is changing but also, importantly, *why*. I meet with patients daily who open up about the manifold reasons they are making choices vastly different from those of prior generations, and I am well versed in how trends in the field are shifting throughout the country.

In recent years, our definition of family has gone through a metamorphosis. The white picket fence, a heterosexual cisgender couple that becomes parents in their early to mid-20s, and a dog are no longer the one-size-fits-all family. Different iterations and varying timelines have evolved and become common: two mothers, two fathers, blended families, single parents, fewer kids, parenthood in middle age, or the choice to be childless.

Long gone are the days when most babies were born to women in their early 20s. Since the 1970s, as more women have become highly educated, participate in the workforce, and aim to establish solid careers, the age at which they have their first child has risen steadily. Between 1972 and 2023, the average age of first childbirth rose from 21 to 27.5, and in 2022 the US Census Bureau reported that the median age of first birth had reached 30. These numbers differ city by city, with the average age of first birth in Manhattan at 31 and in San Francisco at 32. In Italy and Spain, the average age of first birth is 31.6, and in South Korea it is 33.4, so these are trends that have taken hold across the globe.

Women with college degrees have children an average of seven years later than those who do not, as many of them choose to back-burner family planning while they focus on their education and professional advancement. Women outnumber men in college, law school, and medical school, which is an astounding achievement . . . but women's ovaries did not get an extension to account for all those years spent in the library, classroom, hospital, or boardroom! Women in medicine, incidentally, have the highest rates of infertility at one in four because of the length of training in medical school, residency, and possibly fellowship. For this growing cohort of women, any treatment that handles eggs or embryos outside of the uterus can be a compelling offering.

According to Yale anthropologist Marcia C. Inhorn, author of *Motherhood on Ice: The Mating Gap and Why Women Freeze Their Eggs*, as more women become educated at significantly higher rates than men, they experience a mating gap because there are not enough suitable male partners for them. Some of these women are getting married later and then may experience age-related infertility that leaves them turning to ART, while others choose to buy themselves time by freezing their eggs as they continue to look for a partner, and still others choose to become single parents. A large NYU study exploring the various reasons why women freeze their eggs came to a similar conclusion as Inhorn, as nearly 80 percent of respondents reported not being able to find a suitable partner with whom to have children. In my practice, it is quite common for patients to tell me, sometimes with a tone of defeat and other times with acceptance or self-assuredness, something along the lines of, "Jaime, I just can't settle for a man who in my heart I know I don't want to spend the rest of my life with. I'm not looking for perfection, but I know this isn't good enough." Egg freezing or other interventions afford them the option of single parenthood or more time to look for a suitable partner.

We are living longer, yet another reason that delayed parenthood has taken hold. One hundred years ago, the average female lifespan was 58, so having children in one's 20s was especially prudent. Now, the average woman will live until 81. My patients who are having children in their 40s may not be around to meet their grandkids, but the likelihood of living into their 80s or beyond means they can raise their children into adulthood. Our lifespan has extended, but our ovaries have not kept pace, so those who opt for children later in life may turn to ART.

Many people are choosing to delay children for financial reasons. Three out of five Gen Zers (individuals born between 1995 and 2012) and millennials (those born between 1981 and 1996) cite the cost of childrearing as their reason for waiting to have kids, choosing to have fewer children, or not having any. According to the United States Department of Agriculture (USDA), a middle-income family of four will pay about $233,000 to raise a child from birth to age 18, a number that varies by state but which is steadily growing. That is not including the expense of college, which on average costs about $32,000 per student per year. Building a nest egg can take time, and back-burnering parenthood becomes even more compelling for those with access to fertility benefits. Furthermore, 18 percent of millennials report delaying their plans to have children or deciding to have fewer children because of the need or anticipation of the need to take care of aging family members.

People are also increasingly taking their time to settle down, if they do so at all. A swipe-left mindset has transformed dating, as a plethora of possibilities are at millions of dating app users' fingertips. Engaging with multiple potential suitors simultaneously has become the norm, and commitment to any one person can be perceived as banal and restrictive. Why pursue a relationship if there's the possibility of something better just a swipe away? The swipe-left mindset of being noncommittal and wanting to explore all options is not limited to people who date online, as a casual hookup culture has taken hold across numerous demographics in place of relationship seeking and relationship building as primary goals.

This "what if" and "just in case" outlook extends beyond dating. Millennials want options in all aspects of life, including reproduction, and Gen Z has shown similar trends in terms of reluctance to commit across the board. I've had patients, for example, who go into marriages fearing divorce and want a Plan B for having kids at the ready, such as frozen eggs, should they find themselves single again after their childbearing years.

In the 1960s, 72 percent of American adults were married, a statistic that decreased to 50 percent by 2021. In 1970, the average age of marriage in the United States was 20.8, and by 2018 it had jumped to 27.8, with couples, in turn, having children later as well. While unmarried people are less likely to have kids, married couples are also having fewer children or choosing not to have children at all. According to the Pew Research Center, the average number of children in the US family has declined from three in the 1970s to two in 2020 and even lower—to 1.5—for women with a GED or higher. Also, according to a Pew survey, the proportion of adults in the United States younger than 50 years old without children who are unlikely to ever have children grew from 37 percent in 2018 to 47 percent in 2023.

While I cannot draw a straight line between these changing family dynamics and the increase in fertility preservation measures, I can tell you, as someone who has listened to thousands of women and couples opine about fertility plans, that there is a significant correlation. As people get married later, or not at all, and have children later, or choose not to have children right now but want to keep that option open, they are increasingly utilizing what modern medicine has to offer in the realm of fertility.

The fluidity of the concept of gender is another factor affecting people's family planning, particularly as Gen Z ascends into reproductive age. According to a survey administered by the Centers for Disease Control (CDC) in 2023, the number of young adults identifying as transgender quadrupled between 2014 and 2021. The variations of gender are not limited to transgender or cisgender, but also include nonbinary, genderfluid, demiboy, demigirl, and genderqueer. Less than 1 percent of Baby Boomers identify as nonbinary, while 3 percent of Gen Zers do. Society is certainly making strides as gender fluidity is destigmatized and accepted, and we are also making great strides on the medical front in helping couples without the required opposite gametes, or individuals of any gender identity, be able to build a family. There is an uptick in fertility treatment among people who are choosing to freeze their gametes before transitioning in order to maintain the possibility of having genetic children in the future. For example, I have had female patients who, before undergoing surgery to remove their ovaries, freeze their eggs, and I have had male patients freeze their sperm before transitioning to female.

According to a 2024 Gallup survey, more than one in five Gen Z adults identify as LGBTQ+. Since Gallup first measured sexual orientation in 2012, the percentage of respondents identifying as lesbian, gay, bisexual, transgender, queer, or some other sexual orientation besides heterosexual jumped from 3.5 to 7.6 percent. As of 2019, 63 percent of LGBTQ+ millennials were considering starting or expanding their family in the years ahead, a statistic that underscores the rise in ART as a path to parenthood for same-sex couples who lack the opposite gamete.

In 2023, the American Society for Reproductive Medicine (ASRM) updated the definition of infertility to be blind to sexual orientation, gender identity, or relationship status. The previous definition limited all but heterosexual couples from using medical insurance to access costly fertility services. For LGBTQ+ couples and aspiring single parents of any sexuality or gender who needed to access benefits for medical treatment to fertilize gametes, paying out of pocket for treatment made building a family unattainable. Many insurance plans refer to this updated definition in order to determine coverage, and many states—like the 22 states and Washington, DC, that have infertility coverage laws in place—use this definition for various mandates so more people can access fertility services.

The COVID-19 pandemic also left an indelible imprint on the field of fertility. As soon as the acute phase of the pandemic subsided and hospitals were able to accommodate elective procedures, egg freezing soared. Between 2020 and 2022, the Society for Assisted Reproductive Technology (SART) reported a 72 percent increase in egg freezing cycles. My own practice exploded around that time, with a 30 percent increase in those seeking egg freezing. That rise is attributed, in part, to people taking personal inventory during an uncertain chapter, shifting their priorities, and also having the time and flexibility to go through various treatments. I recall many of my patients opening up about a newfound awareness of their mortality and the goal of focusing on building a family. For many, a desire not to be alone was at play so single parenthood beckoned. "I know with certainty now that I really want to be a mom and there is no good reason to wait," one patient in her 30s told me after she had spent years in my office unsure if she was ready to pull the trigger. Some of my patients turned to ART post-pandemic because their newfound ability to work from home made them more optimistic about their ability to have better work-life balance if remote work and modified hours were still intact when they became a parent. Rates of egg freezing increased not only in the United States but globally and did not show signs of slowing down after the pandemic had ended. The United States saw an approximately

40 percent increase in egg freezing from pre-pandemic to post-pandemic, and in the United Kingdom that number jumped to 60 percent.

Not long after the pandemic, *Roe v. Wade* was overturned in 2022, ending federal protection of abortion rights. Since that case, *Dobbs v. Jackson Women's Health Organization*, 12 states have banned abortion rights, leaving many people unsure of how reproductive healthcare access could further be impacted. In another significant post-Roe decision, the Alabama Supreme Court declared in February 2024 that embryos created through IVF are considered human beings, so destroying them is considered wrongful death. This new landscape, with reproductive access making headlines and becoming increasingly politicized, has had reverberations in all aspects of reproductive rights.

While political discourse and recent legal decisions put some procedures in women's healthcare in jeopardy, the fervor and conviction of women wanting to control their reproductive lives has never been more evident. For many, such rulings have been a wake-up call that all kinds of reproductive freedom cannot be taken for granted and that while some rights are being curtailed or dismantled, there are other treatments, like egg freezing, through which women can exert control. We talk about reproductive rights more as they are being taken away, and as the conversation is pushed to the forefront, many women are choosing to take action.

Patients in my New York City practice often come in for egg freezing with a "because I can" attitude, a sense of agency they are excited to use, now more than ever, as they see reproductive rights being truncated throughout the country or feel an existential threat to women's health. They are motivated to plan for their reproductive futures in a way they may never have taken as seriously or as proactively but for restrictions and bans taking hold. In some states, there is a heightened interest in egg freezing over embryo freezing because fetal personhood, the legal term at the heart of many contentious issues pertaining to reproductive rights, does not apply to unfertilized eggs. Many patients are also giving more thought to where they may store their gametes because which state they choose is increasingly relevant to, for example, the disposition of an unwanted embryo.

A significant factor in the changing landscape of family planning is the proliferation of employee fertility benefits, not just infertility benefits. Remember when start-ups and tech companies outfitted their offices with free food, nap pods, and ping-pong tables to help entice and retain millennial workers? Now, employers are increasingly offering wellness benefits, including coverage that makes fertility treatment more accessible and affordable to millions.

As early as 2014, Facebook and Apple began to expand fertility benefits for employees, offering egg freezing for nonmedical reasons alongside coverage for adoption and surrogacy. In recent years, significantly more companies began to offer coverage for treatments including IVF, egg freezing, and gestational carrier services (a.k.a. surrogacy). In 2016, only 2 percent of companies covered egg freezing, and in 2020, almost one in five large US employers (19 percent) offered egg freezing benefits to their employees. Nearly 800 companies worldwide now offer some type of family-building benefits, including Walmart (the largest employer in the country), Amazon (the second largest), Disney, Starbucks, and Meta. In some industries where competition for top talent is high, like law and finance, employee benefits for egg freezing or IVF coverage have become standard, all the more so at top-tier firms. Employees in all demographic groups, regardless of ethnic background, gender identity, or relationship status, are using such benefits and report that this type of coverage is top of mind when considering any career changes.

Increased coverage is also a game-changer for students earning professional degrees, like those in medical school, law school, or on the long road to earning a PhD. Women wrestling with student loans and increasing debt may have previously found the cost of egg freezing unattainable, whereas now their universities or hospitals may offer coverage that makes all the difference for their reproductive futures. By affording younger patients whose fertility has not yet dipped the ability to freeze eggs, success rates have risen dramatically. Some insurance companies will cover the cost of medications leading up to egg freezing even if they do not cover the actual procedure. Additionally, there are now egg share programs popping up that allow women to freeze their eggs for free provided they donate a percentage (usually half) to an egg bank or a clinic.

Finally, the drop in global fertility rates is impacting the utilization of reproductive technologies. In 1800, the average woman gave birth to seven kids, and now it is less than two. In 2022, the European Union reported its lowest level of live births since 1960; approximately 3.88 million babies were born, marking the first time the number fell below 4 million. All European countries, with the exception of Monaco and the Faroe Islands, reported total fertility rates less than 2.0. Canada and the United States also reported declining fertility rates, with Canada reaching a record low in 2023 of 1.3. In South Korea, the total fertility rate (TFR) is 0.72, meaning women there are having less than one child by the end of their reproductive years. Japan's TFR fell to 1.2 from 2.13 in 1970. In some parts of the world, in response to fear that replacement rates are dipping below where they need to be in order to sustain the economy, fertility treatments are being offered by the government. In just three years, from 2020 to 2023, the number of eggs frozen in South Korea jumped to 100,000 from 40,000 because the government covers much of the cost. As many countries grapple with the long-term consequences of fertility rates dipping below replacement level, reproductive technologies may continue to play a pivotal role in helping people overcome fertility challenges—and possibly helping reverse these concerning population trends.

Bottom line: Science has advanced, the world we live in has transformed, and the choices we make have changed dramatically. Women are delaying child rearing for diverse reasons that run the gamut from financial to political to sexual in nature. This has impacted the prevalence of fertility treatment, whether for preventative reasons or because as women wait longer to give birth, age-related infertility and other gynecological pathologies inevitably increase. I have been in private practice for 15 years, and I have yet to see any two patients with the exact same fertility journey making the same choices for the same reasons. The entire landscape of reproductive medicine has changed over the course of my career so far. Getting educated about the latest options for fertility treatments at various stages of life has never been more relevant, pressing, and liberating.

CHAPTER 2

Modern-Day Family Building

I VIVIDLY REMEMBER sitting in Mr. O'Sullivan's class in the 1990s, my 13-year-old classmates and I listening to him as hormones raged inside our developing bodies. We had already learned, in sixth grade, about periods, wet dreams, masturbation, body odor, and pubic hair. In seventh grade, it was a rite of passage to learn about sex. We were lectured about condoms, STDs, the birth control pill, and diaphragms. We giggled, we squirmed, and we learned a thing or two, mostly about safe sex. Mr. O'Sullivan did his best to scare us into believing that if we had unprotected intercourse we would likely pick up a myriad of infections like AIDS, gonorrhea, syphilis, chlamydia, or herpes. Or, worst of all, we'd get knocked up as a teen and scarred by an STD at the same time. Even though AIDS was the leading cause of death for all Americans ages 25 to 44 years old in 1994, the curriculum in my middle school touched only on heterosexual sex, and the primary messaging was, understandably for teens, how to avoid pregnancy.

To this day, I can close my eyes and recall my friends and I cringing as Mr. O'Sullivan demonstrated how to slip on a condom over a banana and the faces we made mimicking vomit when he showed us slides of critters on genitalia infested with crabs and scabies.

Times have changed, but too often, what we learn about reproduction is still old school. Far too many of us still don't know the basic facts about our bodies, let alone about the latest advancements in reproductive medicine. A sperm and an egg still need to connect in order to make an embryo, which can become a fetus and then ultimately a baby; that much remains true. But the ways in which those gametes can make their way to one another, and what can happen after they do, have transformed so much that it's time to update what we used to call, in my generation, sex ed.

I am certainly not advocating that we dial down our efforts to teach young people about safe sex, or that we inadvertently imply they can throw caution to the wind beneath the sheets. Teen pregnancy has declined significantly over the past 30 years, a trend that I very much hope continues, thanks to an uptick in education, access to contraception, and likely increased screen time and isolation, too. At the same time, however, it makes no sense to me why young people learn about breast buds, menstruation, and contraception, but not about the fact that a woman's ovaries throw up a big middle finger at your plans for them starting in the early 30s. People, especially young women, deserve to be informed not just about how *not* to get pregnant, but also the nuts and bolts of how *to* get pregnant, both with and without help from modern science.

Biology Blind Spots

Every summer, I run an internship program for high school seniors, primarily young women, who are accepted into college premed programs. These ambitious young adults already have impressive CVs and plans for their careers, but I am consistently struck by how little they know about their own bodies. Here's a sampling:

> » How many holes we have down there is frequently a stumper. Answer key: The one you pee out of (urethra), the one you poop out of (anus), and then the third is the vaginal orifice.
> » They assume women could get pregnant until menopause and had never heard of perimenopause.
> » Almost none of them know that egg quality declines. They think the eggs a woman has at 20 are just as good as the eggs at 40.

» Miscarriages are mostly a big black box to them, "something that could happen when the pregnancy is off," without any understanding that egg quality may be a factor.

» They know egg freezing exists and has grown in popularity from social media but had never given thought as to why someone might utilize it. (After spending a week with me, their social media algorithms change so they get more egg freezing content in their feeds than they ever bargained for!)

» Most know they want children but have not pondered when it might be ideal to build a family given their plans for long-term education. Not one student has ever thought about a fertility plan, and the general idea of planning ahead for a family is foreign to them. Though they have spent significant amounts of time planning for college and future careers, they think having a family will just happen.

» They do not know that cancer, as well as other diseases, conditions, or behaviors like smoking could impact fertility. Although they have taken and excelled in high school biology, they do not know that certain genetic mutations could lead to infertility, or that preconception genetic testing could help couples avoid passing on certain inherited conditions to a child.

I am not judging them in the least, especially because I remember being like them. I am embarrassed to say this, but I will admit that I did not even know what an egg was or how ovulation worked until I got to medical school! When I had a rotation on the OB-GYN floor, I learned that our fertility is finite because there is nothing women can do to make more eggs. In my residency, when I was rounding the corner toward 30, I really grasped my eggs' inevitable destiny of crapping out on me, but by then I was already standing close to the edge of my fertility cliff.

We can and must do better than that for the next generation. There is a huge gap in understanding everything that happens to a woman's body between puberty and menopause. (It is only recently that people are learning about the ins and outs of menopause, from perimenopause to hormone replacement therapy—a long overdue development.) How fertility starts and how it ends are important milestones, like bookends on our fertility shelf, but a heck of a lot happens in between. I am slowly making headway by teaching in various schools, including at my daughters' all-girls school in New York City. My girls were mortified when I showed up to their class with props, but I believe young people should know that the eggs they have inside their ovaries are precious commodities. The decisions they make—or neglect to make—have life-altering ramifications. Fertility cannot be taken for granted because one day, sooner than most women realize, their eggs will tap out. I do not believe in fearmongering, but I do believe in awareness of cold hard facts and want people to understand what various fertility journeys may entail.

The Building Blocks: Female and Male Gametes

Reproductive cells called gametes, egg and sperm, are the most basic components of procreation. Most women are born with two ovaries, two fallopian tubes, and one uterus. The ovaries are where the primary reproductive hormones, estrogen and progesterone, are made. Housed within the ovaries are eggs, each one encased in a follicle that serves to protect, nourish, and develop them. Unlike men, women's gametes can never regenerate and are finite in supply. A female embryo has peak egg reserve at around 20 weeks gestational age, and then a decline begins in utero. The train leaves the station before you take your first breath and cannot be slowed down. The average female baby is born with roughly 1 to 2 million eggs, which may sound like a lot, but the stockpile, called ovarian reserve, continues to diminish. By the time puberty occurs, women are down to about 350,000 eggs. Even when you are not getting your period, whether because of pregnancy, breastfeeding, or hormonal birth control, egg loss is not paused. It's not just egg quantity that declines. Egg quality is also on a fast tumble downhill starting at around age 30. You know how they say nothing in life is certain except death and taxes? I have an addition to that maxim: Death, taxes, and menopause—when eggs, estrogen, and your period disappear, if you live long enough.

Most males have two testicles, which is where sperm is produced, and a penis. They also have other structures that support the production and maturation of sperm, such as the epididymis, vas deferens, and a prostate. Testosterone, which is produced by the testicles, promotes and maintains the production of sperm and contributes to male secondary sexual characteristics such as male hair patterns, voice deepening, and increased muscle mass. Unlike women, who are born with all the eggs they will ever have, men produce millions of new sperm daily for most of their lives, and that production is happening 24/7. From production to ejaculation is about 70 days, during which time the sperm develops from a germ cell to a mature sperm, traveling from the testicle to the epididymis, on to the vas deferens, to the ejaculatory duct and then to the urethra and beyond. If there's an egg in its path after ejaculation, the sperm may fertilize it and start the process of forming an embryo. Men do not have an abrupt end to their sperm production, but as they age, the chance of their sperm fertilizing an egg in a way that leads to a healthy pregnancy goes down significantly. This is because aging leads to a decline in sperm quantity, motility, morphology (shape), and ejaculate volume.

The Menstrual Cycle

This may be more science than you bargained for, but I think women should know the basics about their menstrual cycle, as this is part of the process through which we lose our eggs on an ongoing basis and the same process that allows us to become pregnant. The menstrual cycle can be divided into four phases: the follicular phase, ovulation, the luteal phase, and menstruation. The first two parts are devoted to growing, developing, and releasing the egg, while the second two are about nurturing an embryo if one is present.

The follicular phase, also called the proliferative phase, is dominated by FSH (follicle-stimulating hormone) and estrogen. This is the phase in which growth takes place for the follicle, egg, and uterine lining. On average, this phase is 12 to 14 days, but it can vary in length from as short as five days to as long as several months. It is this fluctuation that contributes to variable menstrual cycle length.

For most women, one egg is released from the follicle every month in a process called ovulation. Triggered by an increase in LH (luteinizing hormone) from the brain, the surge indicates that the egg is ready for prime time, meaning it has gone through the necessary development to accept sperm if there should be a swimmer hitting the bull's-eye. Approximately 36 hours after the LH surge, the egg is released, completes the second stage of development, and is swept up into the fallopian tube. Even though only one egg is typically ovulated, with each cycle, many eggs are lost. Think of it as a monthly race, with a bunch of eggs vying to be selected as the winner that achieves ovulation. That group of eggs is called a cohort, and those that don't get the winning ticket to be ovulated are then cast aside. Rather than getting another chance to enter in any subsequent monthly races, they deteriorate. For the winning egg, if sperm is present, fertilization can occur. Unfortunately, most of the eggs that women ovulate are abnormal and unable to create a healthy pregnancy. As we age, the percentage of those abnormal eggs increases, making it harder to conceive, let alone conceive a healthy pregnancy.

The luteal phase, also called the secretory phase, is dominated by progesterone. The follicle which previously housed the developing egg becomes the corpus luteum. The corpus luteum is responsible for producing the hormones that maintain the uterine lining that is needed if an embryo implants. The luteal phase should last for approximately 12 to 14 days. If pregnancy does not occur, the corpus luteum will break down, estrogen and progesterone levels will decline, and the uterine lining will shed, which is a period, a.k.a. menstruation.

The length of the menstrual cycle is the first day of your period to the day before your next period. While sperm can live for up to five days in the female reproductive tract and the egg will live for 12 to 24 hours post-ovulation, the days you can get pregnant each month are limited. Knowing your cycle length is important information when trying to conceive because it will allow you to time intercourse and increase the chance of pregnancy.

Getting Pregnant the Old-School Way

Conceiving via heterosexual intercourse, what I'm referring to as the old-school way, is a process that should ideally work like this: When a penis is inside the vagina, ejaculate containing sperm makes its way through a woman's cervix to the uterus, through the fallopian tube, where an egg can be fertilized and create an embryo. The egg would have to physically be there in order to meet up with the sperm, so it has to have been ovulated, meaning released from a follicle within the ovary, and then picked up by the fallopian tube, an event that happens approximately once each month for a woman. The egg lives for up to 12 to 24 hours after it has been ovulated, so there's a tight window for the egg and the sperm to connect when each is in prime shape for fertilization. As women get older, even if they are still ovulating and menstruating, their eggs become increasingly abnormal, so conceiving becomes more difficult. Before the age of 30, a woman's chance of getting pregnant is, at most, 25 percent each month, and then after age 30 chances go down to 20 percent each month, in the best-case scenario. Women over age 40, in ideal circumstances, are looking at a 5 percent pregnancy rate each month. As time goes on in each of these age brackets with failed attempts, the chances get even lower because a smaller percentage of healthy eggs is present. It's a highly inefficient process to begin with, and then aging can add on another layer of difficulty.

If fertilization occurs, hairlike structures called cilia that line the inside of the fallopian tubes pulsate, helping to move eggs, sperm, and eventually embryos through the tube. About three to five days later, if an embryo exists, it should reach the uterus and hopefully implant. By the time the embryo reaches the uterus, it has gone from two cells to hundreds of cells. Here it will grow and divide, becoming an advanced embryo, a fetal pole, a fetus, and then a baby.

Infertility

As I explained in Chapter 1, the definition of infertility was recently updated by the ASRM to no longer assume that it is a heterosexual couple having unprotected intercourse for a predefined amount of time that is struggling to conceive. The meaning of this term can vary, as the World Health Organization (WHO) and the CDC still abide by a definition that disregards the option of single parenthood, assumes the people who want to build a family have opposite gametes, and maintains that a woman in her early 30s should try for a year before seeking fertility treatment. Regardless of the definition that the medical community uses to refer to the inability to get and stay pregnant, women need to know the factors at play.

We know, as well we should, that smoking harms nearly every organ in the body, particularly the lungs and heart. We are well versed in how drugs can harm our brain, that too much fast food can clog arteries, and that sleep and exercise are critical. How about what may impede fertility—did you ever learn about that? Age is the most significant cause, but there are other contributing factors. I'm not suggesting a pop quiz on endometriosis, polycystic ovary syndome (PCOS), fibroids, or tubal disease, but we should all know that infertility is a disease that may very well affect us at an inopportune time. Just as some people who never smoke a cigarette can develop lung cancer, unfortunately, others may experience infertility at a young age without a clear reason or warning sign. We do not always know why some ovaries stop working prematurely, but genetics is often the culprit, so knowing about your mom's, grandmothers', aunts', and sisters' fertility journeys is worthwhile, as it is possible that aspects of yours may mimic theirs.

Various conditions and diseases can affect fertility, such as cancer and cancer treatment. Even if medication or a surgical procedure is not directly tied to the gametes, you can be rendered infertile. Up until 10 years ago, the majority of young adult patients with cancer were not offered the opportunity to freeze their eggs or sperm, or to create embryos, prior to treatment. Nowadays, only 50 percent of oncologists discuss fertility preservation with their patients who are diagnosed with cancer during their reproductive years.

I was diagnosed with breast cancer at age 41, when I had already had my two daughters. I was fortunate that my surgical oncologist discussed egg freezing with me in case I wanted the option of having more children, because the treatment to cure my cancer or the timespan it would take would likely destroy my fertility. I chose not to, as I was not going to try to have any more children, but am grateful for that conversation and the options that were at my disposal. I would like our nation's health curriculum to illuminate for young people all the reasons we can't take fertility for granted, but it's also in physicians' offices where a dialogue about fertility is essential. Patients should be informed about how various diagnoses may affect fertility and, more importantly, what they can do about it.

In Vitro Fertilization

In vitro fertilization, known as IVF, is a go-to treatment for many causes of infertility that brings an egg and sperm together in a lab. If any embryos are created, one or more can be transferred back into a uterus to develop. This treatment, which is covered in depth in Chapter 5, has evolved more than the iPhone since its inception and is one of the most effective forms of ART. Since IVF was discovered in 1978, it is estimated that 13 million babies have been born using the technology to date.

Third-Party Reproduction

Family structures may vary—a mom and a dad, same-sex parents, a single parent, and other configurations—but the actual conception of a child requires opposite gametes, an egg and a sperm, from a genetic woman and man, respectively. Once fertilized, those gametes need a home where they can develop into an embryo, which is what takes place in the uterus. The source of the gametes and of the uterus that carries an embryo can also vary;

when eggs, sperm, or embryos are donated or a gestational carrier helps carry a pregnancy, it is referred to as third-party reproduction. There are numerous factors to consider, the details of which are covered in Chapter 6, but here are the basics.

For same-sex female couples, eggs and a uterus are typically in supply (or oversupply, as there can be four ovaries and two uteri in same-sex female couples), but a sperm source is needed. A donor sperm can address this. Same-sex male couples are typically missing two out of the three fundamentals, eggs and a uterus, so a donor egg and a gestational carrier (also known as a surrogate) are required.

Becoming a single mother by choice has increased in popularity over the last decade. There is limited large-scale data available about the number of women choosing this path to motherhood nationwide, but anecdotally I can confirm that to be the case. In my practice, the numbers more than doubled during and post-pandemic as more women decided that not having a partner will not hold them back from becoming a parent. In order for a single woman to become pregnant, she needs to have a sperm source. My oldest patient who became a single mom was 46 and did so via donor sperm and IVF.

Men can also choose to have children on their own using an egg donor and a gestational carrier. While single fatherhood is significantly less common than single motherhood, more men are coming into our office to achieve parenthood on their own.

Genetic Screening Panels

Perhaps you learned in high school biology class about dominant and recessive traits, like how likely it might be for a child to have blue eyes based on their parents' possible gene combinations. Remember those Punnett square diagrams that helped determine the probability of inheriting various traits, or Mendel crossing peas to analyze inheritance patterns? Genetic testing has evolved so radically over the past 20 years due to advancements in technology, with implications that extend far beyond hypothesizing about eye and blood type as we did back then. Now we can use genetic testing to help create families without passing on a myriad of devastating conditions.

Carrier screening panels are blood tests designed to show if you carry an abnormal variant of a gene which, in select cases, could increase your risk of passing on a deleterious genetic disorder to your future children. In recent years, the number of inherited conditions that we can test intended parents for before getting pregnant or during pregnancy has expanded exponentially. Due to the expanded availability of such panels, more people are undergoing these tests, making it easier than ever to gather critical genetic information.

Given that the panels are identifying recessive mutations, carrying one abnormal copy of the gene will almost never have an impact on an individual. In fact, before undergoing such a test, you would have almost no idea what you carry and its potential impact. However, if both genetic sources are found to carry the same genetic mutation, there is a 25 percent chance of passing that condition on to their children. If the offspring inherits the same mutated gene from both parents, then they will develop the disease associated with that mutated gene. If the parents or genetic sources are both carriers, many couples choose to undergo IVF in order to perform genetic testing on an embryo. This allows for gathering critical information preconception, and avoids the possibility of conceiving a pregnancy affected with a serious genetic condition (such as cystic fibrosis [CF], Tay-Sachs, or sickle cell), which could lead to a significantly compromised life for the child or untimely death.

For those who undergo embryo freezing or IVF to achieve pregnancy, embryos can also be screened for chromosome number before they are transferred back into the uterus. Embryonic genetic testing is the process of analyzing an embryo before implantation to identify chromosomal imbalances or specific gene disorders. This testing has been around since 1990, but it has evolved significantly and can now screen all 46 chromosomes with a high-resolution technique that leads to more accurate and thorough results. As people are having children later, their aging gametes are more likely to be released with the wrong (aneuploid) number of chromosomes. Rather than having 23 chromosomes, they may contain 22, 24, or any other number that can lead to an abnormal embryo, miscarriage, or serious health issues. If preimplantation genetic testing indicates that an embryo is abnormal, it would not be recommended for transfer into the uterus. Confirming that an embryo has the correct number of chromosomes before implantation leads to higher success rates for a healthy pregnancy.

Egg and Embryo Freezing

Oocyte cryopreservation, the scientific term for egg freezing, allows women to pause their biological clocks by extracting, freezing, and storing their eggs. After eggs are extracted, they can remain on ice in a lab indefinitely. If a sperm source is selected in hopes of creating an embryo, the eggs can be thawed, fertilized, and resultant embryos transferred back into the uterus.

More people are also utilizing embryo freezing as preventative medicine. Sometimes referred to as embryo banking or embryo cryopreservation, this procedure requires both an egg and sperm, gametes from a biological man and woman. Those people can be a couple, or either gamete can be secured from a donor. Once eggs are removed from the ovaries, they are fertilized with sperm to create embryos, which then grow for up to a week in a lab; those that survive are frozen. These embryos can be thawed for implantation into the uterus in a short time frame, many years down the road, or never. I will delve into details of these particular modes of fertility preservation, egg and embryo freezing, in the next two chapters.

It has been 47 years since Louise Brown, the first IVF baby, was born. Just like knowing what year we landed on the moon (1969) or when women got the right to vote (1920), I think we all should remember the year when IVF transformed the way humans can procreate (1978) and gauge how far we've come with the advent of egg freezing, embryo freezing, genetic testing, and more. The first great success of IVF was a triumph of medicine; in the decades since Louise Brown's birth, reproductive medicine has advanced even further.

Whether you do your learning in the classroom, at a physician's office, or with this book, I hope that it's clear that how *not* to get pregnant is only one piece of the reproductive puzzle. Just like Cinderella's gown and carriage, the gift of fertility is transient. Before modern medicine stepped in, too many people were not even invited to the ball. The clock does not strike precisely at midnight, as each of us have varying biological clocks, but our fertility will vanish before most of us have half of our lives left to live. Science can jump in as the fairy godmother, but only if you know what the offerings entail and have a plan to set yourself up for a fertile future.

CHAPTER 3

Wear Sunblock and Freeze Your Eggs or Embryos

WHEN I WAS A TEEN, my friends and I baked in the sun while doused in baby oil. Now we know that my baby oil saturation habit was dangerous (not to mention pretty dumb) because the sun's damaging rays can lead to skin cancer. These days, we wouldn't head to the beach without throwing sunblock in our bag, and those of us who want to avoid a sunburn (and wrinkles) are vigilant about applying and reapplying sunscreen. Just as there are preventative steps we can take to protect our skin from a burn or cancer—sunblock, shade, long sleeves, a hat with a wide brim—so, too, do protective options exist for our ovaries.

Oocyte cryopreservation, known as egg freezing, allows women to stop the clock on aging eggs by extracting, freezing, and storing them for potential fertilization in the future. My hope is that just as we instinctively slather on sunblock on a sunny day, more of us will start thinking of egg freezing as preventative medicine in consideration of what may be coming down the pike as our ovaries age. Obviously, sunscreen can be bought at the corner store and sprayed on in 10 seconds, while egg freezing is a costly, time-consuming, more burdensome procedure. But the option of preserving younger, higher-quality eggs, especially as women are having babies later, can be life-changing. Nothing's guaranteed; just as you may wear sunblock and still get a burn or even wind up with skin cancer, not all women who freeze eggs have successful outcomes. Nonetheless, medical advances like egg freezing are highly successful in allowing us to keep the option of having genetic children before infertility inevitably kicks in.

Celebrities on Fertility, Fears, and Freedom

Science has proven the efficacy of egg freezing, but if it takes some A-listers to help me make my point that it is worth considering as preventative medicine, then by all means, let's hear from them. While I am not recommending we trade science journals for TikTok videos, I am acknowledging that celebrities and so-called influencers can be significant factors in eradicating stigma and leading to wider cultural acceptance of egg freezing. I admit that their candid regrets and victories throughout their unique reproductive journeys may be a bit more compelling than the latest dense research papers.

The following is a subset of published remarks from well-known women:

HALSEY (SINGER/SONGWRITER): "When I tell people that, they're like, 'You're 23, why do you need to do that? Why do you need to freeze your eggs? . . . I'm fortunate enough to have that as an option, and I need to be aggressive about protecting my fertility [and] about protecting myself."

RITA ORA (SONGWRITER, ACTRESS): "I think it's amazing the technology we have now to really take control of our destiny. I've always wanted a big family, and my doctor actually said to me, 'I think you should freeze your eggs' when I was in my early 20s. I'm 26 and I know some people might be like, 'Wow, that's so young,' but I just really wanted to be safe."

MINDY KALING (ACTRESS): "I wish that every 19-year-old girl would come home from college and that the gift—instead of buying them jewelry or a vacation or whatever—is that their parents would take them to freeze their eggs. They could do that once and have all these eggs for them, for their futures . . . to focus in your 20s and 30s on your career, and yes, love, but to know that when you're emotionally ready, and if you don't have a partner, you can still have children."

EMMA ROBERTS (ACTRESS): "I did freeze my eggs eventually, which was a difficult process. But I started opening up to other women, and all of a sudden, there was a new world of conversation about endometriosis, infertility, miscarriages, fear of having kids. I was so grateful to find out I was not alone in this. I hadn't done anything 'wrong' after all."

OLIVIA CULPO (MODEL, ACTRESS): "I am going to freeze my eggs so that I can have babies when the time is right for Christian [and me], . . . It's an insurance policy. It's exciting."

SLOANE STEPHENS (ATHLETE): "As a professional athlete, especially as a female professional athlete, you know your time is limited. . . . Family planning relies on the woman to either stop her career or plan to adopt or have a surrogate, so you have to be super proactive in whatever you decide is best for you and your family."

LOLO JONES (ATHLETE): "I just kept thinking I will meet my husband and things will all work out. . . . Well here I am almost 10 years later, and it hasn't. . . . Nothing has scared me more than feeling like I'm running out of time to have a family."

SHANIA BHOPA (TIKTOKER): "My intention wasn't to promote egg freezing but was to open up dialogue on fertility planning. Why can't we start thinking about fertility earlier and open up the conversation so that you can plan and be open-minded to other ways of conceiving? . . . The Disney effect around women is that we're going to live this serendipitous life and hopefully at the snap of our fingers get pregnant when we want to, when we're ready, when it's 'meant to happen.' . . . But then we hit 35, and the truth is, women face a lot of challenges with fertility."

I wish more young men and women knew about the relatively new options in the realm of fertility preservation, including embryo freezing. Even those who may never elect to go down this path should be informed about the advances and the possibilities that exist. Personal reasons for choosing to freeze eggs or embryos could be waiting to find the right partner, establishing one's career, or simply because reproductive autonomy is cherished under any circumstances. Medical reasons might include cancer that affects fertility, ovarian surgery, endometriosis, autoimmune diseases, or genetic mutations. It is far less common to freeze sperm, given that men typically have a constant supply of ample sperm, but when a man is going to undergo chemotherapy, surgery that could impact sperm, or has a reduced sperm supply, freezing is often considered.

#Eggfreezing has gotten more than 117 million views on TikTok to date, a metric that leads me to presume people are seeking accessible information about what egg freezing entails and why it may be worthwhile to consider. I'm not sure they're prioritizing seeking out the most scientifically sound and reliable information when scrolling on social media, but that's what I'm providing here. In this chapter, I will delve into the history of egg and embryo freezing, along with a bit of the science behind it. As always, I will tell it to you straight, including sharing stories from patients, some of whom agree with me that egg freezing is the greatest gift since the invention of the pill, as well as others who feel differently.

From OG to (Almost) Mainstream

The idea of fertility preservation beyond medical necessity is relatively new. In 1978, the birth of Louise Brown, the first baby conceived through IVF, confirmed to scientists that an egg could be successfully fertilized outside of a woman's body. The first babies born using a frozen egg were Australian twins in 1986. This was more than three decades after the first baby was born from frozen sperm, eight years after the first IVF baby, and two years after the first birth from a frozen embryo. So why were eggs the last to undergo cryopreservation? For good reason. The size, water content, and developmental stage at which they are frozen make eggs incredibly susceptible to the formation of ice crystals and resulting DNA damage. Safely freezing *and* subsequently thawing and fertilizing the egg, which is the largest cell in the body when mature, is a very complex undertaking.

Over the course of the next nine years, until 1995, there were only five additional births worldwide resulting from previously frozen eggs. The abysmal success rates initially were due to the nascent slow-freeze and rapid-thaw cryopreservation techniques. A new technique was developed called vitrification, which reduced potential egg damage with flash freezing. In 1999, the first pregnancy and live birth from vitrification occurred in Australia. Since then, cumulative data from around the world has confirmed that the process of vitrification for egg freezing is a significant improvement, with the majority of high-quality clinics achieving 80 percent post-thaw survival rates. From the 1990s until 2012, oocyte cryopreservation was considered experimental by the ASRM and used primarily for young women with cancer whose treatment could harm their fertility or for those facing imminent fertility loss or risk of premature ovarian failure.

Patient POV

Sloane, 29

When I was diagnosed with breast cancer at 24, egg freezing was recommended as an option to preserve my fertility before chemotherapy and radiation. Breast and ovarian cancer has burdened women in my family for generations, so knowing that by freezing my eggs I would not only be able to maintain the option of having kids, but also be able to test embryos in the future to ensure my children would not have the BRCA2 mutation, sounded like an incredible option. I knew very little about the process, but because I wanted children in the future, the decision to move forward with two rounds of egg freezing was pretty easy. I found it to be very manageable, both physically and emotionally, partly because I felt so fortunate that I could do it, had an amazing support system, and had full faith in the team of doctors and other medical professionals who were guiding me.

But for my cancer diagnosis, I don't think I would have considered egg freezing. Now I have a sense of security that my eggs are waiting for me whenever I am ready to use them. As we get into our 30s, I want my single friends who are stressed about the pressure to find a partner and start a family to know that egg freezing is an option for them too! There's such a lack of awareness about the process, so I'm trying to encourage other women to get educated and consider it. I surprised myself at how capable I was to do something that seemed so scary and foreign. I'm stronger and braver than I thought. I'm cancer-free and now I have the chance of becoming a mom, too.

In 2012, the experimental label on egg freezing was removed by the ASRM and the SART, though initially they expressed caution about its use as a measure to guard against inevitable age-related fertility decline. Women could undergo oocyte cryopreservation for purposes of fertility preservation, known as "social" or "elective" egg freezing, giving them autonomy to delay childbearing by circumventing the effects of age-related infertility.

While many hailed elective egg freezing as a significant step, others viewed it skeptically, criticizing that fertility clinics were providing false hope at high fees. There were concerns that use of this new technology could present religious, ethical, and cultural challenges. Some feared that it would pressure women to prioritize their careers once they had the option of back-burnering parenthood, while others worried it would exacerbate the gap in access to healthcare if only affluent women could afford it. Nonetheless, once ASRM gave its stamp of approval to elective egg freezing, the procedure began to gain acceptance.

Most OG elective egg freezers, as I like to call them, were toward the end of their reproductive years, choosing to undergo the procedure as somewhat of a Hail Mary before the window to get pregnant with their own egg had closed. Just like a Hail Mary pass in football rarely wins the game, the OG egg freezers' efforts were met with limited success. The challenge, we now know, was that because the average age of a woman freezing eggs in the early 2010s was in her 40s, egg quality was already compromised. No matter how good the cooling and warming process was to freeze and thaw such a delicate structure, the outcome would inevitably be poor if the eggs were past their prime in the first place. These suboptimal results gave OG egg freezing a bad wrap, but as some younger women with higher-quality eggs began to undergo oocyte cryopreservation, patient outcomes improved.

The proliferation of social media, expansion of employee fertility benefits, the COVID-19 pandemic, and a long-overdue spotlight on women's health were all factors in elective egg freezing taking off, particularly among those who had the means to pay for it out of pocket or who were fortunate to have comprehensive benefits that included fertility preservation. As fertility clinics began to expand nationally, fertility benefits became more commonplace, financing options became available for those whose benefits were limited, and egg freezing parties became part of the cultural zeitgeist. Additionally, social media influencers publicly shared their egg freezing journeys, reducing the previously held stigma about fertility treatment. Urgency to find a life partner or make any life decisions, personal or professional, with one's biological clock in the driver's seat was reduced or, for some, even eradicated.

In my own practice, the narrative changed from a defeated "I can't believe I have to freeze my eggs" to a confident "Why wouldn't I freeze my eggs before my fertility inevitably plummets, especially if I can do it on my employer's dime?" I saw friends come in together with their egg freezing cycles synced so they could share the experience together. The vibe of patients looking down in the waiting room to avert any eye contact was replaced by a sense of camaraderie among like-minded women who refused to be tethered to an immutable time frame for reproduction. I saw a five-fold increase in women undergoing egg freezing in just over five years, from 2018 to 2023. Nationwide data shows an 800-fold increase in the number of egg freezing cycles performed from the early 2010s to the 2020s. With so many younger women taking the plunge, success rates soared. A large study out of NYU in 2022 reported a 70 percent live birth rate for women who froze eggs before 38.

In 2023, the ASRM released an updated version of their "Ethics Opinion on Planned Oocyte Cryopreservation to Preserve Future Reproductive Potential," standing in strong favor of egg freezing as an elective procedure to increase reproductive options, enhance autonomy, promote social equality, and improve women's ability to organize education, work, and family building with less pressure from their biological clock. The statement expressed that because women are inherently disadvantaged with a reproductive window that is narrower than males, expanding this window with egg freezing is a means of leveling the playing field in terms of not just procreation but also with regard to education and the workplace. The ASRM acknowledged the benefit of women not needing to use donor gametes if they froze their eggs, a consideration that could eliminate the cost and complexity of undergoing IVF at a later time. This watershed opinion from the ASRM also recognized the impact egg freezing could have on transgender individuals who might lose their female gametes, families that suffer the death of an existing child, and people who want additional children after unexpected life events like divorce.

Younger Is Better

So what, you may be saying. Good for womankind that this option exists and seems to work pretty well, but why do it? Is having fertility tethered to a biological clock really a risk? Isn't that just how life and our bodies are meant to work? Hitting the snooze button on some eggs requires self-inflicted shots, numerous blood draws, and outpatient surgery—who needs that? Even if insurance covers the procedure, storage for eggs can be an out-of-pocket expense lasting years. Making ends meet can be hard enough without the cost of freezing eggs that may or may not ever be used. Why plan for something that may not be an issue for you and will likely drain your bank account? These are all fair questions that we ought to be asking, and more importantly, questions you need answers to.

I know I sound like a broken record, but women are born with all the eggs they will ever have. Unlike the typical male, who releases 20 million to 60 million sperm in a single ejaculation and then promptly has it replenished by his testicles, women lose millions of eggs before we are even out of the womb. At birth, most female infants have around 1 million to 2 million eggs, and by puberty, the count is down to approximately 350,000 to 500,000. Before we can even use them we are losing them! From puberty to menopause, the decline of eggs continues, at first steadily and then rapidly. Think about a graph with X and Y axes. As your age (X) rises, your egg quantity (Y) drops. By 25, a woman loses nearly 80 percent of her eggs. By 35, the number of usable eggs that are gone jumps to about 95 percent. The unfortunate math does not end there. We are not only losing quantity but also quality, and it is this combination that leads to age-related infertility. This means that at age 38 you will not only have fewer eggs but those that remain are of reduced quality. At 30 you have approximately a 20 percent chance of getting pregnant every month, and by 40 this number has dropped to around 5 percent.

Call me crazy but I think aging is pretty awesome. All the jokes about a midlife crisis or middle-aged misery don't resonate. Other than my knees getting a little creaky and my wrinkles staring back at me in the mirror more prominently than I would like, I feel great and think all the wisdom I've accrued over the years is paying off. When it comes to eggs, however, the equation is quite simple and indisputable: Younger is better. Those are the facts; I am just the messenger. This is why I am ringing the alarm bell to encourage people to think about this option as preventative medicine starting younger, not a last resort once the best of your eggs have decided to peace out.

Patient POV
Kelly, 51

When I was 39 and single, a friend convinced me to freeze my eggs to ease the pressure of meeting someone and as insurance to be able to have kids. Back then, in 2012, egg freezing was not common at all. In fact, it was not something people even talked about. Until my friend mentioned it, even though I knew my clock was ticking, I had an attitude about marriage and kids along the lines of, *Everything will just work out the way it should.* In hindsight, I realize how shortsighted, even ignorant, that mindset was.

Even though there were a lot of doctor's appointments and shots, the process was straightforward, easy, and painless. I did one round and got 23 eggs, which I thought was a success. I started dating in a more relaxed way and met a guy I really liked. Early on, I told him I had frozen my eggs, which I think made it easier for us to have fun and get to know each other without the pressure that if we got serious, we would have to start a family right away. We got married at 42 and came up with a plan before trying to get pregnant. We would use the frozen eggs first, then try IVF again if needed, then use donor eggs, then adopt. That helped us feel confident that no matter how our baby would come, we would build a family together.

We thawed the eggs, made embryos, and two of them were perfectly healthy. One became our miracle son, whom I gave birth to on my 44th birthday. When our son was a toddler, we tried to use the second healthy embryo that we had frozen, but it didn't work. We tried several rounds of IVF when I was 46, which also were unsuccessful. Looking back, I felt confident with my one round of egg freezing but should have done one or two more rounds to increase the odds of having multiple children. I would have if I only knew, which is why I want other women to be educated. We need to be able to make decisions with a full set of information, especially as the process evolves. Still, I'm thankful every single day that with this technology I was able to have a baby at 44.

A large study published by NYU showed that women who froze 20-plus eggs under the age of 38 had a 70 percent live birth rate from thawing their eggs. At the national clinic where I am the Director of Egg Freezing, internal data shows similar rates, with success improving dramatically for younger patients. Research also shows that the younger a woman is at the time of the freeze, the fewer eggs she will need for success after thawing, so one is likely to get a lot more mileage from ten 28-year-old eggs than from ten 38-year-old eggs. Said differently, in order to provide a 40-year-old with similar success rates as a 30-year-old, the older woman would need to freeze about four times the number of eggs. I have a love/hate relationship with skiing, the sport that took out my ACL, but skiing offers a good visual to understand why. In this analogy, every woman hits the slopes. You hop on the mountain and hang out on the bunny hill in your 20s until about age 32. It's just smooth sailing, no bumps in sight, with a slope that is barely noticeable as you gently coast downhill. That is when your fertility is at its peak and it is the easiest to get pregnant. Just as some people find the bunny hill challenging, there are those who will still encounter fertility challenges at a young age due to various causes. (I speak from experience, as my ACL snapped on an easy run!) After the bunny slope, you can cruise on greens for a bit. When you hit around 35, you have graduated to the intermediate runs, the blue ones that have a steeper downhill and some unexpected bumps, just like your fertility. By around age 37, you're up to a double-blue and getting down safely grows even more difficult. At this point, a typical woman might be left with around 25,000 to 35,000 eggs of modest quality, making it more challenging to achieve a healthy pregnancy. You might make it down the double-blue without falling, just as you may hit the bull's-eye fertilizing an egg at this later age, but it is not a foregone conclusion by any stretch. When you hit 40, prepare to nosedive down a black diamond, hurtling down the hill as eggs disappear at a rapid pace. No different than how every woman menstruates or goes through menopause at a different time, this is not a hard and fast timeline. Some women may stay on the bunny slope until their mid-30s, while others are tumbling down double-blacks long before they intend or want to be, but these age ranges are a typical gauge. There is also an avalanche risk posed by cancer and other illnesses that can destroy fertility at any time—all additional reasons we may need that Other Plan B.

Unlike a real ski resort, here there is no off-ramp or cozy nook to hide out drinking hot chocolate; you are stuck on the slopes along with everyone else who has ovaries. Even when you are not getting your period, are pregnant, breastfeeding, or on birth control, you are still on the hill with your eggs in decline. In this analogy, the only way to get off the mountain, to stop the decline in egg quantity and quality, is by freezing reproductive tissue. Egg or embryo freezing are the only technologies that allow women to freeze a cohort of eggs or embryos for possible future use, thereby pressing pause on the inevitable downward spiral. And while it is not a guarantee, it is the closest thing we have to assurance for preserving our future fertility.

In most cases, your body will not send you signals indicating when your egg supply will come to a halt. Using blood tests and ultrasounds, doctors can tell you how many eggs you may get in a retrieval and can estimate how many may be freezable (based on maturity) in that group of eggs. There is no way of predicting if those eggs will be good, bad, or somewhere in the middle, and if you might be able to create one baby, multiple babies, or none at all. With the data from blood draws and ultrasounds, we can compare patients to others in the same age bracket based on larger population studies, but unfortunately we cannot assess if one has high-quality, viable eggs. For example, if I have a 32-year-old patient who I estimate would get between 12 to 18 eggs, with hopefully around 70 percent that are at the ideal stage to be frozen. I would be able to declare that her hypothetical outcome would be age appropriate. Until we do the retrieval, this is all just educated speculation. It is only after we have physically removed and examined the eggs that we have reliable numbers. Many of my patients find this incredibly disconcerting, understandably. In my mind, the lack of insight we have into one's future fertility is all the more reason to plan ahead.

My high-achieving Type A patients typically cannot wrap their head around the fact that when it comes to fertility, there are no goals they can set and then knock out of the park with hard work to tilt the scales toward a favorable outcome. After spending most of their life acing every test in school, crushing it on the athletic field, excelling in the arts, attending prestigious universities, and reaching the highest levels professionally, it is unfathomable to them that they can wind up in their late 30s, with or without a partner, facing limited options because their eggs are already past their prime.

Likewise, my patients who are in excellent overall health often fail to grasp the possible dichotomy between general well-being and ovarian function. How is it that a woman who never misses a checkup, barely catches a cold, eats clean, runs marathons, and does not even drink can suffer from ovarian aging? Early-onset infertility or any other reproductive challenge does not necessarily come with a warning or reflect the rest of your health. I was in excellent health in my 30s, exercised regularly, ate healthy food, and still got breast cancer. That same unpredictability applies to fertility. But there are, thanks to modern medicine, preventative options like mammograms to screen for breast cancer and egg freezing to extend fertility. Just as I believe it's worthwhile to take advantage of preventative screenings, it's a boon to womankind that we can, increasingly with insurance coverage, pause a previously unyielding biological clock.

It astounds me how much time and money people in their 20s, 30s, 40s, and beyond spend trying to halt or slow the aging process. From skin-tightening moisturizer to firming cream, repair serum, eye gel, and laser treatments, women go to great lengths at great cost as they endeavor to turn back the hands of time. They may see subtle changes, but all the lotions, potions, and Botox shots in the world can't erase the wrinkles, fine lines, and lack of collagen that belies our age. (I am also blown away by how much the tween market focuses and spends on skincare, but their motivations are quite different.) I am not critical of these efforts, and as a middle-aged woman, I myself sought out noninvasive antiaging "remedies." What confounds me is how committed and open-minded some women are to slowing down signs of the natural aging process *externally*—willing to try all kinds of gimmicks even while knowing the results may be modest at best—yet will not pay attention to an effective fountain of youth in the realm of fertility.

Egg freezing, which freezes time for our eggs, has proven to be a successful treatment when done at the right time on presumably fertile patients. (If we freeze eggs for someone who is unknowingly infertile, then when eggs are thawed, we would still face challenges.) More and more women seem to be getting the message. In 2012, there were 2,719 egg freezing cycles performed in the United States. In 2023, the latest year for which there is data, there were approximately 40,000 cycles of oocyte cryopreservation performed in the United States. That's more than a 1,300 percent jump in 11 years! As my practice has morphed from women using egg freezing as a last resort to an empowered and liberated first resort, I stand on the shoulders of scientists and clinical teams around the globe that have performed study after study for decades to prove that egg freezing is a safe, viable, and successful procedure. These trailblazers helped open a world of reproductive options, allowing a diverse population to access various paths to parenthood. It is, I believe, incumbent upon physicians to build on these successes by making it standard of care to offer a fuller picture of fertility to their patients (and their parents, when appropriate) so even more people can consider joining this reproductive revolution.

Patient POV

Dana, 36

As I was approaching 35, my gynecologist opened my eyes to the fertility limitations that come with age. I had just gotten out of an eight-year relationship, during which time I thought I didn't want children, but when it ended, I realized that maybe I did. I'm a dancer who has dedicated my whole life to my job, which has taken a toll on my body, relationships, and more. When my doctor suggested that freezing my eggs would keep open the possibility of having children one day, I decided to give myself that chance. Freezing my eggs was one way I felt that I was giving myself options, helping me feel like a whole person beyond my career and beyond my new relationship status as a single woman. I am still unsure if I will ever have children or use the eggs I froze, but I do not want to look back with regrets. My experience was successful, but it was much more difficult than I expected in terms of the physical toll and how long it took me to recover. I was lucky to have two other women in my life going through it at the same time as me because I think it's so important to have a community to support you.

Banking on Embryos

Embryo freezing, also known as embryo banking or embryo cryopreservation, is undoubtedly one of the most game-changing lab technologies. It requires both an egg and sperm, gametes from a biological man and woman. Those people can be a couple, or either gamete can be secured from a donor. Once eggs are removed from the ovaries, they are fertilized with sperm to create embryos, which then grow for up to a week in a lab. Thereafter, those that survive that weeklong lab stint will undergo a biopsy procedure to analyze if the embryo has the correct number of chromosomes before being frozen. Once frozen, embryos can stay on ice indefinitely. Many large-scale studies have demonstrated no impact of prolonged freezing on embryo survival, clinical pregnancy, implantation, miscarriage, and live birth rates. When embryos are thawed, they can be implanted in the initial patient or in someone else's uterus.

In the past decade, there have been significant advancements in embryo freezing, embryo biopsy techniques, and genetic testing of embryos. Modifications in treatment protocols and lab techniques pushed single embryo transfer success rates to 75 percent in select clinics. As the technology has improved, the number of embryo banking cycles has risen exponentially in recent years. According to SART, for clinics in the United States, 3,380 embryo banking cycles were performed in 2015 and 13,090 in 2023, a nearly 300 percent increase. It is hard to get an exact figure nationally or globally about embryo freezing specifically for fertility preservation because the statistics are typically lumped together with embryo freezing as part of IVF, but anecdotally I can validate the uptick in embryo freezing purely for fertility preservation purposes in my own practice. There are an estimated 1 million frozen human embryos stored in the United States, and according to the SART registry, that number may actually be higher than 1.2 million frozen embryos. Worldwide, of course, the number of frozen embryos is far greater, with Spain reporting 600,000, 100,000 in the United Kingdom, and 100,000 in Australia. Again, not all of these are intended for fertility preservation, as these numbers include surplus embryos that were created during IVF cycles as well, but clearly it is a procedure that has become more commonplace.

Although embryo freezing has existed since the 1980s, it was not until recently that it made headlines when the Alabama Supreme Court ruled that embryos created through IVF should be considered children. We have yet to see this ruling's long-term impact on fertility treatment in Alabama or elsewhere, and as a physician I am not here to weigh in on what is already a politically and religiously charged landscape. I do, however, believe that now more than ever we have a responsibility to get educated, so let's dig in.

As early as 1971, and well before embryo freezing in humans, embryos of mice, cattle, rabbits, horses, and monkeys were frozen and thawed. Not until 1983 were scientists able to successfully freeze a human embryo, and the first baby born from a two-months-frozen embryo came into the world in 1984 in Melbourne, Australia. In the years that followed, doctors in countries including the United States, Israel, the Netherlands, and Britain were able to successfully freeze human embryos, and hundreds of thousands of babies have since been born from the process.

Embryo freezing, which preceded egg freezing, started as a way to preserve surplus embryos that were not transferred in a fresh IVF cycle. In the early days of IVF, when numerous embryos were transferred to increase the likelihood that at least one would take, many patients ended up with twins, triplets, or more. Who can forget "Octomom" Nadya Suleman, who gave birth to the first surviving octuplets in 2009? (Fun fact: Suleman is now a grandma!) If some embryos could be frozen and then thawed for later use, the thinking went, not every embryo would need to be transferred simultaneously, and high-order multiple pregnancies would decrease. In 2013, the ASRM released a practice guideline that women under 35 with a high-quality blastocyst (advanced embryo) should have only one embryo transferred at a time. Most couples and physicians heed that guideline, opting for a single embryo transfer and freezing any others for possible future use. According to the CDC, in 2022, 85.9 percent of women under 35 undergoing IVF or embryo freezing transferred a single embryo.

Patient POV

Carolina, 31

I miscarried twice in a row, and we now know that the embryos were abnormal. So many friends confided in me about their miscarriages and how it's the unspoken secret women carry—or more accurately, don't carry. I am in an incredibly fortunate position that my husband's work has fertility benefits that cover up to $50,000 in treatment, so we decided to do IVF in order to test future embryos before implanting them.

I questioned if this was like trying to control fate or interfere with what should be a more organic process, especially because I'm *only* 31, so in theory we have a bit of time. But now that science gives us the ability to see what kind of embryo we're creating, giving us the chance to choose a healthy one, how could we not take advantage of that opportunity? I'm not excited about injecting my body with hormones or even the idea of *picking* our baby if we're lucky enough to have that scenario, but after two miscarriages that took a toll physically and emotionally, that seems like a small price to pay.

In many ways, the history of egg and embryo freezing are intertwined, as developments in the freezing and thawing process for each tissue type allowed for improved success rates for both. Just as with egg freezing, in the early days of embryo freezing, a slow-freeze/rapid-thaw technology was used. It worked well on day three embryos, which we call cleavage stage embryos, because they are quite small and do not contain much water. When embryos were transferred on day five, however, at what is called the blastocyst stage, many did not survive the thaw. Results were modest because day five embryos contain a large fluid-filled cavity called the blastocoel, which hinders the proper penetration of cryoprotectants and can lead to the formation of ice crystals. This damages the embryo's delicate structures and reduces viability after thawing.

The slow-freeze/rapid-thaw process for embryo freezing was eventually replaced by vitrification, which minimized ice crystal formation and allowed clinicians to achieve an approximately 95 percent thaw survival rates for blastocysts. In the United States, frozen embryo transfers now make up 80 percent of all transfer cycles; the remaining 20 percent are fresh embryo transfers, with no freezing involved before implantation in the uterus.

People choose to freeze embryos for a variety of reasons. Some patients aim to preserve their fertility because they will undergo cancer treatment or any other medical intervention that can affect their ability to get pregnant or carry a pregnancy. Whether they have a partner with whom they are committed to starting a family or are planning on single parenthood, embryo freezing would be a suitable option.

Others turn to embryo freezing because, unlike egg freezing, embryos offer real-time data on the health and viability of the gametes. This is particularly helpful when one or both partners carry a genetic condition they do not want to pass down to their offspring, like BRCA or CF. Embryonic genetic testing, the process of removing cells from an embryo for analysis before embryo implantation, is also utilized to identify chromosomal abnormalities. The testing has been around since 1990 but has evolved significantly and can now screen all 46 chromosomes with a high-resolution technique that leads to more accurate and thorough results. If an embryo is abnormal, it would not be recommended for transfer into the uterus because it would be unlikely to survive or could lead to serious health and developmental issues.

Some undergo embryo freezing not for medical reasons but for personal ones, like couples that value the ability to have children on their own timeline, without their gametes calling the shots. Perhaps a couple has career aspirations that may hijack peak childbearing years, or they want wiggle room to travel the world. I had a patient who I later found out was delaying pregnancy because of her role in the CIA, and another who got cast in her dream role on Broadway so she postponed family building. Some want to delay the arrival of a child until after they have built a nest egg, especially because housing is so expensive, or they simply want to get used to being a couple living together before adding in the stress of a child. Embryo banking can also be an insurance policy to allow for having multiple children despite advancing age, to enable more years to pass between each child rather than rushing to beat the clock, or to transfer to a surrogate when a pregnancy cannot be carried.

Patient POV

Sonya, 33

My husband and I are deeply in love with each other, and there is no question we want to have a family. We would like to have either two or three kids, but first our plan is to establish our careers. I am on the cusp of a big promotion at a hedge fund, while he is trying to make partner at a law firm. Having kids now could derail our professional ambitions, so we want to give ourselves a bit of time.

Knowing with certainty that we both want kids together, we decided to freeze embryos. As of now, the timeline we have in mind for parenthood is about four years from now. We haven't yet decided if we'll try to conceive naturally or immediately thaw the embryos that will have been made with younger eggs and are already tested. There is something incredibly reassuring about having the extra time to put family-building on hold on so many levels. I go to the office every day with exceptional grit and passion because each day that I can work toward my goals without needing to also balance parenting is a gift.

Don't get me wrong—when the time comes, I know there will be a difficult balance as there is for all working parents. But I'm not ready for it just yet. It's about economic stability but really about so much more. We have worked our whole lives to build careers that we value. I just need four more years to feel like I'm not throwing that all away in order to make my dreams of parenthood also come true.

Couples are now flocking to fertility clinics as a part of their premarriage checklist. Just as they might meet with a financial planner to lay out assets, goals, and a timeline for buying their first house, talking to a fertility specialist helps gather critical information from each person and create a joint road map. If the goal is to one day not just buy a home but also fill it with children, which it is for many, then communication and preparation along with help from a practitioner are essential. You would not start house hunting until you knew your budget and desired location, right? Before starting a family, too, it is ideal to know what you are each bringing to the table in terms of gametes, genetics, hopes, and more. The course of action may need to change as we uncover possible obstacles or as priorities shift, but having such a plan is critical nonetheless.

In my practice, when couples come in before their "I dos" to discuss plans for creating a family, I often say to them, "No BS, tell it to me—and to each other—straight. Where are each of you on the kid thing? How many do you want and what is your time frame?" For some, it is too abrasive an approach, but I believe it is part of how I do my job well because without raw honesty, we cannot make suitable decisions about the future. It is also how, around 30 percent of the time, we discover that there are major disparities in what each half of a couple has in mind. One half may want kids pronto while the other is barely committed to the partnership, let alone to parenthood. In a couple of rare instances, I've suggested that couples rethink their relationship. (Yup, I'm that blunt.) Most of the time we use this dialogue as a jumping-off point to review their medical histories, family histories, and talk about how many kids they might want and when. We run diagnostic blood tests, such as ovarian reserve tests, genetic carrier screening panels, and semen analysis. These tests do not indicate if someone is fertile or infertile, but they do shed light on how the various pieces of the fertility puzzle are functioning, individually and as a couple. For example, if a semen analysis shows very low sperm count, it does not mean a man will not be able to father a child, but that is a challenge that might require surgical or medical intervention. Such tests also illuminate for couples any recessive genes they may carry, information that is helpful to have at the outset rather than when once they are ready to start trying. Advancements in preconception panels provide information about hundreds of genetic mutations, which means both you and your sperm source can know what you each carry and if there are any concerning overlaps before a pregnancy occurs.

Patient POV

Renee, 38

I have the infertility trifecta: fibroids, endometriosis, and one fallopian tube from an ectopic pregnancy. After 14 years with my husband, during which time we were holding off on starting a family, we decided to take advantage of the amazing fertility insurance that my company offered by freezing embryos. My only out-of-pocket expense was the co-pay for medication.

I was 36 when we did the retrieval, and I naively assumed it would be a one-and-done situation. It took three cycles to get five embryos, which really surprised me. I didn't expect the emotional hiccups, the feeling of *What's wrong with my eggs?* It's like March Madness except instead of teams, it's eggs and embryos being eliminated at every stage. By the end, I was sore, bruised, and so over getting injected. It definitely put a halt to my life for a week, but now I can breathe knowing we have embryos on ice.

I am going in for my transfer in two days! The prep for the transfer was, in my opinion, a bit more uncomfortable than the prep for egg retrieval. While I wasn't constantly injecting myself, the nausea and hot flashes from letrozole left me agitated and uncomfortable. Hopefully it is all worth it though. I wish I could say I felt ready, but I think that for me, taking the leap will always be filled with a bit of fear—and that's OK. I am lucky to have doctors I trust and to have embryos in the freezer. It is so important and empowering for women to take ownership of our lives and our bodies.

Risks, Cost, and Unrealized Hopes

I may be nicknamed the Queen of Egg Freezing, but that does not mean I believe egg freezing is right for everyone. A 46-year-old who wants to build a family can count on me to champion her decision, but not via egg freezing. It is not just about age and success rates when I help a patient evaluate if oocyte cryopreservation is the right course of treatment. Everything we do comes with a potential downside—in life and in medicine—so it is incumbent upon us to weigh risks and benefits. Ideally, medical professionals would guide patients through the process, exploring pros and cons, side effects, recovery, success rates, and more. This is the standard I hold myself to, but a doctor's transparency, authenticity, handholding, and integrity cannot be tested on a board exam or graded on a multiple-choice test. As with any medical treatment, patients need to do their homework and make the best decisions for themselves.

Even with extensive research, vetting, and proven safety, things can go wrong with egg freezing. A cycle to preserve fertility can expose infertility.

Egg yields can be disappointing. Not all eggs survive the thaw. Those that do survive may not fertilize. Not all embryos pass genetic testing. Those that are chromosomally intact may not transfer seamlessly. If the transfer is successful, it may still not result in a pregnancy. Not every seemingly healthy pregnancy leads to a live birth. There are countless other issues that can arise, such as uterine abnormalities, autoimmune diseases, hematologic conditions, and pelvic pathology like endometriosis, all of which can prevent even the best previously frozen eggs or embryos from progressing into healthy pregnancies.

To describe the risks of egg and embryo freezing, I use a three-pronged approach: medications, the procedure, and the aftermath.

MEDICATIONS: The majority of my patients over the last nearly two decades are rockstars both in terms of administering their medications and tolerating them. Like professional chemists, they draw up, mix, and then inject themselves with twice-daily shots. Symptoms from the medications are common but fairly short-lived, typically no longer than the latter half of the treatment, which is about seven days. These symptoms may include abdominal bloating, transient weight gain, breast tenderness, mild bruising at the injection sites, temporary allergic reactions like redness at the injection sites, nausea, sleep disturbances, mood swings, increased vaginal discharge, and mild electrolyte disturbances. Most side effects subside within one week, while bloating, weight gain, breast tenderness, and abdominal discomfort may remain present until the period following the egg retrieval begins. Think of the arrival of your period like popping a balloon; it marks the beginning of your return to normalcy as all the hormones keeping any symptoms present get a severe interruption.

Women who have an excessive response to fertility stimulating hormones, as demonstrated by a large number of growing follicles and high estrogen levels, are at risk for ovarian hyperstimulation syndrome (OHSS). Mild OHSS occurs in about one out of three women post–egg retrieval, with symptoms including nausea, bloating, and pelvic discomfort. In select cases, like severe OHSS, the ovaries can become dramatically enlarged, and large amounts of fluid can build up in the abdomen and possibly the lungs.

This can lead to difficulty breathing, dehydration, and severe abdominal pain. While the advent of new stimulation protocols in the early 2010s significantly reduced the incidence of severe OHSS it still affects approximately 2.5 percent of patients. Administering a medication called leuprolide rather than human chorionic gonadotropin as the final trigger to prepare the eggs for maturation and release can prevent OHSS but could possibly compromise the number and maturity of eggs retrieved, so there are trade-offs. Like I said, we always need to weigh risks and benefits, so this is something you ought to discuss with your physician.

THE EXTRACTION: For most patients, the procedure is outpatient surgery requiring conscious sedation anesthesia. After a brief recovery on-site demonstrating the ability to eat, drink, and urinate, patients can head home to take it easy. By the next day, most people are back in the office or doing their regular activities but with modest exertion until the next menstrual cycle. There is, however, a 1 percent chance of excessive bleeding from damage to blood vessels, injury to surrounding organs, or a chance of infection. This number is even lower when the procedure is performed in a clinic with qualified and experienced board-certified physicians, but that still does not mean it is nonexistent.

THE AFTERMATH: Egg or embryo freezing can preserve your ability to have a genetic child at a later time in life, but it is also possible that your hopes of genetic parenthood will remain unfulfilled. You can put a lot of time and money into the process and come out with nothing but debt and grief. You can alter the course of your life, perhaps maxing out credit cards or sticking it out in a job you hate because of the benefits, for a potential that never pays off. The process can falter at many points, like failing to survive the thaw, an inability to be fertilized, or failing to grow as an embryo in the laboratory. In some cases, the embryo grows in the lab, but after the transfer to the uterus there is a negative pregnancy test. We don't always know why. You can do everything right and it can still go heartbreakingly wrong.

In 2023, when the ASRM Ethics Committee deemed elective egg freezing ethically permissible and supported its ability to enhance reproductive autonomy and support social equality, this governing body also reinforced that it is an evolving procedure with uncertainties. Patients need to be informed, and providers need to be forthright about its efficacy, safety, risks, benefits, and cost. They cautioned against labeling the procedure as an "insurance policy for future childbearing" for fear it would perpetuate a false sense of confidence when the quality of one's eggs is unknown. They encouraged more workplace coverage for the procedure but expressed concern about aggressive or even coercive marketing practices. Egg freezing remains a relatively new treatment, so even though offspring born from previously frozen eggs do not appear to have any increased risk of anomalies, compared to babies born via IVF, long-term data is limited. The ASRM reiterates: "Patients considering this treatment must be apprised of these unknowns."

Prospective patients also need the unvarnished truth about cost. On average, egg freezing, not including medications and anesthesia, costs between $7,000 and $12,000, based on facility and location. Depending on the dose of medication required, that cost can increase by $2,000 to $7,000. Once the procedure is complete, storage for the frozen eggs can run about $500 to $1,200 per year, with possible discounts available if you store for a minimum number of years. You may want to consider storing in a long-term storage facility other than at the clinic, as sometimes off-site locations are less expensive. Keep in mind that different facilities have various selling points and prices to match, like digital identification and tracking to reduce the possibility of any mix-ups, automatic real-time inventory, customer portals, security protocols, and processes for retrieving from storage. Also, there is a fee to thaw, which runs another $10,000 to $12,000, and then another cost to transfer, around $4,000 to $7,000.

Freezing embryos can cost you upward of $20,000 plus the cost of medication and anesthesia, depending on the clinic, geography, and treatment regimen. With embryo freezing there may be an additional cost for genetic testing, which can be up to $3,000 depending on the facility and number of embryos tested. When a patient's usable embryo yield per cycle is low, there may be a need for multiple cycles. Once embryos are created and frozen, storage fees are incurred annually, ranging from $500 to $1,200, which especially adds up if they are stored for many years.

Insurance companies are increasingly covering some of these costs. According to a 2022 Mercer study, nearly 20 percent of large employers in the United States (defined as companies with 500 or more employees) cover elective egg freezing. This number increases to 37 percent for large high-tech employers and 63 percent for *Fortune* 100 Best Companies. These numbers have grown substantially in the last few years as companies ranging from Walmart, Target, Amazon, and Applebees to JetBlue, General Motors, and Amtrak compete to attract and retain talent by offering comprehensive benefits. Entire fields such as tech, law, and financial services are shifting their benefits, and other sectors, including healthcare and education, are gradually following suit. Increased coverage has enabled more younger women at the inception of their professional lives, who have yet to build a savings account, the opportunity to freeze their eggs. Nonetheless, egg or embryo freezing remain procedures that not everyone can access, so for some, the cost of owning your reproductive future can be exorbitant.

Patient POV

Paige, 48

I was 35 and single when I decided to freeze my eggs. The catalyst was that I had friends around my age whose IVF attempts were taking a toll on their body or who had miscarried several times, but ultimately what it really provided for me most was optionality. Freezing eased the pressure of dating and really just any pressure on myself in general. Everything became a nonissue for me mentally.

The actual process was a good experience for me. I viewed it as a task I had to focus on hard for two weeks, like a project I needed to get done with success. Not being able to exercise rigorously was probably the hardest part, but I walked a ton, which I felt eased the hormonal effects. I also did acupuncture a lot, specifically during the week of retrieval. I got a lot of eggs, which made the pain I felt after the retrieval worth it. I recovered pretty quickly too.

I never planned on having a baby on my own, so I have not thawed the eggs, but it was still worth it for the peace of mind and optionality. It eliminated the mental gymnastics around kids, timing, and who I did or did not date because wanting to be able to have a baby didn't have to factor into my decisions. I still pay to store them even though I would probably not have kids at this stage, but I value knowing they are available to me if I change my mind.

I have been as forthright as I can possibly be that not all egg or embryo freezing cycles are successful, and there are no guarantees. I do not want to give women a false sense of security that if they freeze eggs they can become mothers whenever they want. The necessity of sperm to fertilize the eggs and create embryos presents another layer of complexity. Is fertility medicine a business aiming to increase its consumer base? It is. And yet I passionately believe that egg and embryo freezing are medical miracles that have transformed the lives of millions for the better. These reproductive innovations give women the option to own their fertility—period. What I have found, over and over again, is that most people almost never regret having done it, even if the process is futile or they choose not to use the eggs. I have had patients get only one egg, while others have gotten 51, and they are equally thankful for having had the option of trying to freeze time for their precious gametes. Knowing they are headed toward infertility, as we all are, but they exerted agency prevents them from living with a *shoulda, woulda, coulda* mindset for years to come.

A Mother's Wish

My girls are my everything. When they were toddlers, a chunk of lollipop stuck in a molar did not faze them, so it was my job to get them to brush their teeth. As they got older, a steady diet of pizza and pasta would have suited them, so it was my job to throw in some broccoli and protein. I can see around corners when they may not be able to, which is why it is also my job to set them up for a fertile future. I have no idea what obstacles will get in their way throughout life, but I hope their biological clocks won't be one of them. It doesn't have to be! We can freeze time, in a way, by preserving fertility.

In my effort to help my daughters experience the boundless joy and privilege akin to the one that I have had as their mom, I hope they will agree to let me freeze their eggs after they graduate from college. They know that as much as I wish I could make middle school mean girls be nice or prevent them from experiencing heartache, I cannot. What I can do, however, is preserve their future fertility so that if they want a family one day, they can hopefully make their dreams come true, unfettered by aging ovaries. They may never want children, or they may have children without ever using those eggs. They may use their frozen eggs successfully or try to use them to no avail. I do not know what the future holds, but I want them to have the ability to shape their own paths based on their minds, hearts, and passions, not their reproductive clocks. What incredible freedom!

Since my girls entered the world, the gratitude I feel for the privilege of parenthood has motivated me even more to pay my gift forward. It is my fervent hope that other women will be inspired to wear sunblock and freeze their eggs or embryos, or take charge of their fertility in whatever way is right for them so they, too, can embark on a wondrous journey of their own from a position of knowledge and proactivity.

CHAPTER 4

What to Expect
When You're Freezing

WHETHER I'VE PERSUADED YOU about the importance of having the Other Plan B intact, you were already planning to preserve your fertility, or you're simply getting informed about what various options entail, this chapter will give you a step-by-step guide for egg and embryo freezing. Before you decide if either is right for you and move forward with treatment, I recommend that you discuss the possibility with trusted advisors, such as your internist or gynecologist who knows the specifics of your health, as well as close friends who can be a sounding board.

If you proceed with egg or embryo freezing, you will need a fertility specialist and a clinic with which they work. They will serve as your pit crew, the team that knows you and your reproductive organs inside and out, as they shepherd you from a consultation to the finish line. Choosing a clinic can be as complex as finding a partner on a dating app. What you see is not necessarily what you get, especially when your first glance may be on social media, where influencers touting one clinic over another are frequently paid for their messaging. Your physician may have a recommendation, but depending on where you live, your options may be limited. Large metropolitan areas tend to have multiple fertility clinics, whereas people who live in more rural areas may have to travel quite a distance to reach the nearest clinic, perhaps even across a state border. At the time of writing, New York City has 43 fertility clinics with 68 locations (and more are popping up), while in the state of Wyoming there are, as of now, none. New telehealth platforms allow consultations across the country, but where one does the actual procedure may be limited by geography.

Not to minimize my expertise or impact, but I am not the most important person on my patients' egg or embryo freeze team. So much of success in the fertility arena is not only dictated by the clinical team but also by the embryology laboratory and the scientists who play a pivotal role. A good or even incredible physician paired with a poor embryology lab far too often leads to a suboptimal outcome. Clinics with both experienced clinicians and high-quality embryology laboratories have more success with ovarian stimulation, egg extraction, the egg freezing and warming process, and the growth of embryos.

When choosing a clinic and lab, consider not only where you live now but where you may plan to live in the future. If you freeze your eggs in Denver but may soon be moving to Houston, for example, make sure you have the ability to send the eggs to a clinic there. If you live in a state where reproductive rights are limited in the aftermath of the demise of *Roe v. Wade* or potentially impacted by the Alabama Supreme Court decision that embryos are to be considered "unborn children," it is worth thinking about storing your eggs or embryos in a different state or with a clinic that has a national network of clinics in many states. Fertility clinics that have national networks are ideal options, given that they have sites in multiple cities and can seamlessly send gametes to sister clinics that have the same freezing and thawing protocols in order to maintain the highest level of fidelity and quality.

As you consider the best team for you, here are some questions you may want to ask, followed by the kind of answers you should be hearing. Keep in mind that everyone's circumstances and resources vary.

How many cycles of egg or embryo freezing does your clinic do each year?
A cycle is akin to a round of egg or embryo freezing, meaning the start-to-finish process from the first shot to the extraction of eggs or creation of embryos. A clinic that does a significant number of both egg and embryo freezing cycles each year is ideal. Some clinics may do thousands each year, whereas others that have fewer physicians and less demand do

fewer. But the idea is that you want a clinic that does both egg and embryo freezing. If they only do egg freezing, then how will you create embryos down the road? If a fertility clinic only specializes in egg freezing, then thawing the eggs and creating healthy embryos may not be part of their expertise.

How many thaws has your clinic completed and what is the thaw rate?
For fertility clinics located in metropolitan areas, where the vast majority of egg and embryo freezing procedures occur, according to seasoned embryologists, at least 100 egg thaws demonstrates comfort with the procedure. Ideally at least 80 percent of eggs should survive the thaw. That survival rate should be even higher with embryos; in a high-quality clinic, the embryo thaw rate should top 95 percent. (Medical websites are not the easiest to navigate for non-MDs, but national data about embryo thaws is posted on the SART website.) In rural areas with possibly fewer patients or when a clinic is newer, these may be unrealistic numbers, but you should still ask how many procedures they have completed and what percentage of those eggs or embryos were viable post-thaw. Trust your gut if it seems like they are experienced and offering solid results, while also referring to the data that is available.

What is your live birth rate from frozen eggs? Of all the eggs that are extracted and then frozen, what percentage lead to babies?
As a general rule of thumb, the success rates for egg freezing should be equal if not better than the success rates for that same-age patient for IVF. While you are not comparing apples to apples because they use different technologies and there are different types of patients using each procedure, comparing the same age groups provides a useful indicator of success rates and lab competence.

Who performs the procedures? Are they board certified or board eligible?
While there are many procedures that physician extenders (e.g., physician assistants, nurse practitioners) can do, an egg retrieval should be performed by a licensed physician. After four years of a residency in obstetrics and gynecology, fertility specialists spend another three years in

fellowships learning how to extract eggs and transfer embryos. You want someone with this level of training to perform your egg retrieval, which will take place on a date dictated by your ovaries. If it will be a physician, is it yours or the doctor who is on call on the day that your ovaries indicate it is go time? If it is the latter, that may be perfectly fine, but it is information you should know ahead of time, particularly because some clinics have a "doctor of the day" model, with a rotation of who is on call, rather than having access to your own physician. Are all the doctors in the group board-eligible or board-certified reproductive endocrinology and infertility MDs? Only physicians who complete and pass both written and oral board exams receive board certification. Being doubly board certified is a big deal; it means a practitioner is trained as an OB-GYN in addition to fertility. (Take it from someone who has taken a lot of exams: There is no harder test than the reproductive endocrinology and infertility boards!)

Will you, my doctor, be the one making decisions about my treatment plan, dosing, when to extract, and how many cycles to do, or am I assigned to the person on call depending on my timing?
Oftentimes decisions need to be made urgently. When that is the case, who will be the team member weighing in on what your ovaries or uterus need? Understanding who will be making the final call surrounding protocols, including daily medication dosing and egg retrieval timing, is of the utmost importance. These may seem like simple tasks, but it is actually the art of fertility medicine. The science happens in the lab, and the medication dosing and timing is the art. You want the *artist* who knows your specific case to be making the decisions on your treatment.

If I need to get in touch with a clinic, how do I do that?
This may not be a deal-breaker when choosing a clinic, but it is still good to understand up front if you will be communicating via a patient portal, email, phone, or any other method. If you have a question, how do you get in touch with someone and how quickly will you hear back? I have

found a two-way patient portal is best because it allows for fairly constant and consistent communication between doctor and patient, but not all practices or clinics offer that.

After an egg retrieval, who follows up with me about the results, and what's the ballpark result I should hope for?

Following an egg retrieval for either an egg or embryo freezing cycle, you will likely receive a postoperative call from a nurse to see how you are feeling. The hope is that you are not in pain, you are eating and drinking, and you are using the bathroom (just urinating is sufficient). You should also expect to receive a call from your primary physician (even if they did not do your procedure) or be contacted to schedule an in-person appointment to review results from the egg retrieval, including how many eggs were retrieved and how many were frozen. Typically, 70 percent of the eggs extracted should be at the appropriate stage of development and therefore able to be frozen, so ask what the norm is for any particular clinic.

Where do your eggs or embryos go after they are frozen? What are the safeguards and backup systems to ensure the eggs or embryos are safe?

After the eggs or embryos are extracted and frozen, they can either remain in an on-site lab, or they may be shipped to a long-term cryo storage facility. If they are shipped off-site, you should know where the facility is and how much notice you need to give the clinic if you want to use them in the future. Ensuring that your embryos are frozen in a licensed, skilled facility with multiple backup systems is essential. Storage tank malfunctions, while infrequent, have occurred, destroying thousands of embryos and people's plans for future fertility along with them. How are the specimens labeled, are systems automated or manual, and what is the process for retrieving embryos when you are ready? Ask questions to find out if the facility has ample safeguards, electronic and physical, to ensure the security of the eggs. Newer storage companies have introduced automated robotics that allow for 24/7 remote monitoring of frozen eggs or embryos by using digital trackers, which are highly advantageous.

Do you offer support services to patients going through egg freezing, such as mental health, acupuncture, or nutrition?
I think it is worthwhile to ask about additional support services because mental health providers, acupuncturists, and nutritionists can collectively help you have the best outcome. (In Part 2, I cover more on what, specifically, these alternative treatments may add.) If no such services are offered, it is not a deal-breaker, but it might be a consideration if you have several options.

How much does it cost? Are there grants or financing programs?
Cost is a huge consideration as you choose a clinic. You should be well-versed on your employer's benefit plans before embarking on this process. Make no assumptions about whether or not your company covers egg freezing, as the offerings are changing rapidly across the board, whether at massive corporations or small businesses. Cost varies based on factors like geography, type of clinic (private versus academic), and multipackage options, like whether you are interested in more than one cycle.

In many cases, you pay for your egg freezing up front and, if your employer offers any fertility benefits or insurance coverage, you would be reimbursed later. Medications are often a separate fee paid directly to the pharmacy. Annual storage fees are generally waived for the first year and then run about $500 to $1,200 annually thereafter. Most fertility centers have finance departments that should be able to help you, including where to access loans or grants and how to navigate insurance benefits. I also recommend researching payment plans, loans, and financing through companies like www.futurefamily.com. Grants may be offered if you are dealing with a specific illness or have other unique considerations. Some patients pay for this investment in their future by using credit cards, even though interest rates are typically higher than loans.

It is beneficial to gather information from a variety of sources, such as the fertility clinic, your referral source, and national registries like SART and CDC, both of which have begun to collect more data on fertility preservation in recent years. Clinics are required to maintain internal data, so asking for it is par for the course; if they are reluctant to share such information with you, that is a red flag.

Your fertility doctor should be forthright with you that there are no guarantees with egg or embryo freezing. There is no way to ensure that the procedure will yield the results you seek. If a doctor declares that under their care you are undoubtedly going to have success, you should be skeptical. On the flip side, if your physician is overly negative and thinks you are wasting your time, I would take seriously what they have to say but consider if that mindset of defeat before even beginning will make the process more challenging. I currently have patients with whom I've been quite clear that their eggs have seen better days, but I am very optimistic about the fact that they will achieve parenthood with donor eggs. Find the right fit for you both in terms of expertise and energy. If you're on the fence, I recommend a second opinion.

I love team sports because I am an avid fan and a mom of athletes, but also because I cherish the fact that when you are part of a team, nobody wins alone. The same goes for a successful egg or embryo freezing cycle. The physician cannot do it without the nurses, medical assistants, embryologists, and care coordinators. Not a day goes by without me leaning on members of my team in order to provide patients with the best treatment outcomes. My door is always open (which can be annoying to my colleagues when I'm listening to Taylor Swift at top volume) because creating an atmosphere of collaboration and welcoming suggestions from all members of a team boosts us all. Bravado does not go far in fertility, or in any area of medicine for that matter; I would be wary of any physician who does not seem like a team player.

Patient POV

Ava, 34

I got married at 29, and the marriage ended when I was 30. I knew I wanted to have kids, and I wasn't on the path I wanted to be on anymore. Life throws you curveballs, but I was lucky to work at a company that covered egg freezing. Finding the right time was a challenge because I travel for work a lot, and I wanted to run the New York City marathon before I had to start giving myself shots, so I timed it around that.

I'm a pretty tough cookie, a self-reliant, I-can-handle-anything kind of person, but I underestimated the emotional and physical toll this would take. The entire process was much harder than I expected. The most important advice I would give anyone going through this is to have a support system lined up. Other than having someone pick me up from the egg retrieval, I did it completely alone, and that was a mistake. It's a lot to go through, especially alone. I also should have arranged to work from home or given myself a little break from work altogether.

I now feel incredible peace of mind that I extended the timeline for becoming a parent. I move through life more relaxed and go on dates without fear and pressure hanging over my head. Knowing that having a husband who had an affair and left the marriage isn't the end of my story is liberating. Life is different than how I planned it, but now I have options and flexibility, and I can have a completely full life with or without finding a partner.

Once you have selected a practitioner, you'll set up a consultation. Egg or embryo freezing consultations and follow-ups include a lot of talking, with questions about your medical history, including surgical, gynecological, reproductive, and family history. It is also an opportunity to convey how many kids you may want, what your ideal timeline would be, and any other relevant details as you plot out a possible fertility journey. In my office, I go deep with my patients on their hopes and dreams, both short and long term. That is partly because I cherish my connection with my patients, but also because it is good medicine. Your doctor should be your partner who is "in it" with you as together you chart your course. Other topics for your initial visits might include when certain medications like birth control or GLP-1s (e.g., Ozempic, Mounjaro, etc.) must be stopped, the right time to undergo the process with a two-week commitment, and how you will finance the procedure. A consultation or follow-up also includes a vaginal ultrasound and blood draws to test egg quantity, the presence of infectious diseases, blood type, blood count, and thyroid levels. This is all important information as you and the provider gauge how many rounds of egg freezing you may want or need based on the data gathered and what your target goals are.

Team Embryo vs. Team Egg

You may also use your consultation to discuss egg versus embryo freezing for you. My daughters often ask me, half-joking, but still hoping to hear the answer they want: "Which one of us do you love more?" Like my response to that ridiculous question, when it comes to egg versus embryo freezing, I am a proponent of each for different reasons. I spend a significant amount of time counseling patients as they make this sometimes difficult decision, and these are some of the primary considerations.

Once a woman freezes her eggs, they are hers and hers alone to do with as she pleases. She may choose to thaw and fertilize them with sperm in hopes of becoming a parent when the time is right, donate them to enable another woman to conceive, or never use them at all. It is 100 percent her call. I cannot emphasize enough how badass I think it is for a woman to step into the driver's seat of her reproductive future, calling the shots on when she uses her eggs, with whom, and how. Although there are no guarantees, her reproductive future is hers to navigate, untethered from her biological clock and from any particular sperm source.

An embryo, on the other hand, is the joint property of both parties who created it, excluding donors, and therefore both have equal rights about its use. If two partners freeze an embryo and then proceed to break up, neither of them can use the embryo without the other's permission unless agreed to in advance or determined during a separation or divorce agreement. So, for example, if one person wants to become a single parent with the embryo while the ex-partner refuses to give access to their shared creation, a contentious legal showdown may ensue. Such challenges affect same-sex couples as well if their relationship dissolves.

In one case that made headlines, actress Sofía Vergara sued her ex, Nick Loeb, and the reproductive center where they made embryos in a seven-year battle about what would happen to their embryos post-breakup. Ultimately,

Vergara was granted a permanent injunction preventing Loeb from using the embryos without her explicit written permission. This is a high-profile example of how vital it is to have legal agreements in place prior to creating embryos and how contentious it can become when a relationship dissolves.

We cannot ignore the sobering statistic that around 50 percent of marriages end in divorce, not to mention how many premarital relationships do not last. While most marital assets can be divided somewhat equally, once a sperm and egg come together, there is no "unscrambling" the egg, so it is vital to have legal agreements in place prior to creating embryos.

Embryo freezing is the clear winner when it comes to data, because only once the egg and sperm come together can we apply any kind of testing to glean information about DNA, viability, and more. The egg on its own cannot be tested, so we know nothing about its quality, ability to be fertilized, or capacity to create a genetically normal embryo, whereas an embryo presents an enormous amount of information quickly. Once embryos are tested, only the most viable or desirable are used for implantation. I am a marathon runner, so I think of it this way: Eggs are running the 100-meter dash, and they can make record time, but we are not so sure how they would do in a longer run. Embryos are training for a marathon, and they get a check-in after they have run a half before they continue to the finish line. Once they show they can survive to the blastocyst stage (days five to seven) in the lab, they are more likely to make it the whole distance. Then, at the 20-mile marker, the embryos get another big push forward when genetic testing can confirm the appropriate number of chromosomes. The marathon isn't complete until a healthy delivery ensues, so there is still a long stretch to go, but by mile 20 the embryo is set up for success.

My overall take: Eggs win for autonomy and embryos win for real-time data and for the additional vetting by virtue of having survived in a lab. If I see a patient in her 30s who knows she wants to become a single parent in the next year, I would give a thumbs-up to embryos. If she does not yet know her time frame for parenthood, I would suggest eggs. For couples with concerns about passing on a hereditary condition, embryos are advantageous for their ability to be tested for specific genetic mutations that either both or one partner may carry. For a patient who is in her 20s or early 30s and just wants to buy time while looking for a partner, my vote would be eggs. I prefer embryo freezing for couples who are getting married in the near future or who are already married but want to postpone parenthood—if both partners are on the same page in terms of their commitment to each other and to building a family, including the timeline. Disagreeing on the timeline can be a red flag, so please do not kid yourself by saying, "We're 100 percent on the same page about having a family, except I'm ready now and he wants to wait a few years." That is not the same page. It can be hard to accept, but you do yourself no service if you're not honest with yourself and each other.

As a woman, as a divorcée, and as a physician who has seen many women get an exceptionally unfair hand in terms of their reproductive journey, I have a bias toward egg freezing for younger single women and for couples whose union is shaky. More often than not, when it comes to frozen embryos after the demise of a relationship, the woman is on the losing end of this equation. If a relationship falls apart, the embryos get taken down along the way, which can leave the female partner without access to her younger eggs once they are fertilized with her ex's sperm. Men will make sperm for almost the entirety of their lives, so in most cases they can maintain the opportunity to have children as they age. A woman's fertility runway is shorter, so she's back to square one but with older eggs, which may diminish her options for biological parenthood. This is not always the case, but a woman's biology leaves us more vulnerable to infertility with each passing day, so freezing eggs is one way to keep options open.

Regardless of specific circumstances, in general I believe that because life is unpredictable, Team Eggs is a safer bet. No joint custody, no two-person decisions, just sole proprietary ownership while gametes can remain frozen in time until utilized. Good eggs frozen in a good-quality lab will remain eggs with potential when they are thawed. By "good" I mean eggs that are mature at the time of retrieval and extracted from a woman in the prime of her reproductive years. We have to wait until the eggs are thawed and fertilized to find out if any of them can lead to chromosomally healthy embryos that are capable of creating a pregnancy. In my view, that's a small price to pay for having the freedom to pivot and move down any reproductive path as life unfolds. There are also fewer ethical concerns like embryo disposition, and egg freezing is less costly up front than embryo freezing.

Some patients ask to do both embryo and egg freezing in one round of ovarian stimulation. I do not think it is wise to play on two teams; I advise patients to pick one for each game. In order to get the best outcome, eggs should be evaluated in a cohort, as a group in their entirety. When a patient asks about combining egg and embryo freezing in one cycle, like splitting half of the eggs for one and half eggs for the other, it reminds me of my daughter doing her homework while watching TV. Do not do a half-ass job—not with your homework and not with your fertility. One fertility preservation cycle at a time, egg or embryos, is ideal.

Patient POV

Molly, 37

I was dead set on my plan of becoming a single mom by choice at 32. I closed myself off from meeting someone, decided I was comfortable being single, and just wanted to become a mom. I guess I felt old, which seems insane now. My doctor, who knew I really wanted to meet someone and get married, said: "You just haven't met 'him' yet, but you might. If this was 10 years down the road, we might be having a different conversation, but maybe right now isn't yet the time to become a single mom by choice."

She suggested I freeze eggs, and ultimately I agreed. It was a very emotional process for me, mainly because I felt like the first person in my family or among my friends to do it and because so much about it was completely unknown to me. By the time we did a second round of egg freezing, I had a whole different mindset. I knew what to expect and found it empowering that I was proactively taking steps to preserve my fertility. After two rounds, I had 18 frozen eggs.

I had thought I needed to decide my life plan by 32, but that was short-sighted. I fell in love, got married, and four years after I froze my eggs, my husband and I made embryos. We now have a daughter, and I am pregnant with our second child. My egg count was low for my age, so had I waited even a year longer, I might have been too late. I feel incredibly fortunate and want other women to find out as much information about their bodies as early as possible. Not to be cheesy or trite, but knowledge is power.

Nuts, Bolts, and Hormones

If you decide to move forward with either egg or embryo freezing, make sure you tell your doctor all medications or supplements that you take, both prescribed and over the counter. In most cases, oral contraceptive pills or other hormonal medications like the patch, ring, injectables, and implants need to be discontinued at least one month before egg freezing can be initiated. IUDs, on the other hand, do not need to be removed because the ovaries can be stimulated and eggs extracted without interference. Medications that increase the risk of bleeding or anesthetic complications or impact the production or binding of hormones, such as spironolactone, must be discontinued.

All fertility treatments start with your period. Like a gun blast that kicks off a horse race, your menstrual cycle signals the beginning of the process, and the growth of your follicles, which contain your eggs, are off to the races. On day two or three of your period, it is time to begin injectable fertility hormones that are usually administered twice daily over an average of nine to 14 days to stimulate the production of multiple eggs. We don't want just one winner in this race; we want to promote the even growth of all follicles, which is promoted with hormones at the beginning of the cycle. Such hormones are synthetic versions of the hormones our brains make, FSH and LH, which help an egg grow, mature, and ultimately ovulate monthly in a natural cycle. In most cases, you ovulate only one egg each month, but by stimulating the production of multiple eggs with fertility hormones, the number of eggs released can dramatically increase. The dose of medications and the way they are mixed together depends on factors such as egg quantity, age, medical history, and in select cases, previous fertility treatments.

Many people ask if the hormones have side effects or increase the risk of cancer. Patients report feeling bloated and crampy, but there is no definitive evidence of long-term risks, nor is there a proven causal relationship linking an increased risk for gynecologic and breast cancers with IVF and fertility medications. For patients diagnosed with cancer, there has been no evidence that fertility medication advances the cancer stage, promotes cancer spread, or increases the chance of future recurrence.

The hormones are self-administered as subcutaneous (meaning the fatty tissue under the skin) injections twice a day for 10 to 12 days at hypernormal doses to allow several follicles and the eggs within them to grow and mature together at an even cadence. I think of it like a marathon with a pacer who keeps everyone together. When stimulated by hormones, the follicles and the eggs inside are tracked on a daily (or every other day) basis with ultrasounds and hormonal blood tests. The goal is for all the eggs to go through growth, development, and ovulation as a team, so the race is watched regularly to make sure no one egg is taking the lead. Once a patient starts the hormones, intercourse is strongly discouraged due to risk of pregnancy and ovarian torsion.

What one chooses to do with the eggs after retrieval has no impact on the process of ovarian stimulation, including hormonal injections, morning blood work appointments, and ultrasound checkups. Whether eggs will be frozen or the goal is to create and freeze embryos, most women go to the clinic every two to three days in the morning for blood work and ultrasound. Women with higher egg counts may need more frequent checks. These visits typically last no more than 30 minutes. While no one likes to get their blood taken before their morning coffee, for most patients the monitoring is pretty painless. It typically takes about 10 to 12 days for follicles to increase in size and for estrogen levels to rise as the eggs they house develop. Younger women may require lower doses of stimulatory medication and have a shorter time frame before egg retrieval, while older patients frequently require higher doses of hormones and a lengthier stimulation process. Estrogen levels and follicle measurements together provide fertility doctors with data to make decisions on when to modify medication doses, how frequently to monitor the patient, and when the ideal time for the extraction procedure will be. Your fertility clinic should be providing you with daily communication regarding your medications and when to return to the office. Giving yourself too much or too little of the hormones or missing an appointment can impact the outcome of the egg or embryo freezing cycle, so take this process seriously.

For both egg and embryo freezing patients, the same data points— follicle size, levels of estrogen and progesterone, and length of stimulation—

determine when is best to administer the final injections, called trigger shots. Whether you are instructed to take one or two trigger shots is dependent on your treatment regimen. Although they are typically self-administered, some people may hire a nurse or ask a partner or friend to pitch in because the trigger shots are the most time-sensitive and important. Additionally, the dose of such medications will vary depending on factors such as your baseline LH level, your peak estrogen level, your AMH (Anti-Müllerian hormone, which is a surrogate marker for egg quantity) level, your follicle count, and your BMI.

What is most important when it comes to trigger shots is timing. You must take the shots at the exact time you are told. Being early, late, over-sleeping, or waiting until a meeting ends can result in cycle failure or cancellation. I tell patients to set two alarms and have a friend set one, too, so as not to miss the right timing for trigger shots. If I had a nickel for every patient who called in a panic about being 20 minutes late for their trigger or panicking that the needle they need for the injection is missing, I would have my girls' college tuition covered. No, 20 minutes won't make or break your success, but being several hours too early or too late for the procedure can tank the outcome. (Don't get me wrong: Being on time is ideal!)

Until the ovaries and estrogen levels give the go-ahead, it is unclear what day the retrieval will be, so don't expect to definitively know when the main event will occur more than two days before the procedure. When follicles typically reach around 17 to 18 millimeters and the patient's estrogen reaches the appropriate level, it is time for the egg retrieval. Most fertility clinics perform the egg retrieval 35 to 36 hours after the trigger medications are administered. To allay any anxiety and ensure you're ready to go on the day of retrieval, I recommend setting more than one alarm and having everything laid out the night before as you might have done before the first day of school as a kid.

In the majority of fertility clinics across the country, the egg retrieval is performed in an operating room under anesthesia to avoid pain and ensure there is no movement during the procedure, which could increase the risk of bleeding. You will arrive, having fasted from the night before, approximately 45 minutes before your procedure at either the operating room that is part of the clinic, a hospital, or another facility. Your surgical team, consisting of a nurse, anesthesiologist, embryologist, and the physician performing your procedure, will get you prepped before the surgery. This prep includes putting on a surgical gown, checking your vital signs, and reiterating the plan for your eggs or embryos. Whether the clinic uses conscious sedation, deep sedation, or general anesthesia, you should not feel pain during the procedure. In fact, you probably will not remember any of it when you wake up in the recovery room. As with any surgery, vital signs (heart rate, blood pressure, and oxygen saturation) are monitored continuously.

After the patient falls asleep, typically lying supine, the surgical team will place the patient's legs in stirrups and will clean the vagina before starting the egg retrieval. A vaginal ultrasound is used to guide a needle that traverses the vagina, punctures the vaginal wall, and enters the ovary. Once the needle is inside the ovary, the physician pierces each follicle (the shells that hold the eggs), draining the fluid inside. There is a suction device connected to the needle; the follicular fluid is aspirated by the needle, the eggs detach from the follicular wall, and they are ultimately sucked out of the ovary into a test tube. This procedure is repeated until all of the follicles are drained. In the operating room, it is not possible to see the eggs inside the follicles or even in the tubes. Only when the eggs are inside the lab can they be officially identified, cleaned, and analyzed for their stage of development and viability by the embryology team. As the physician moves from follicle to follicle, the embryologist is at a microscope in the lab, shouting out the egg count. While most procedures take no more than 30 minutes, when there are more follicles or the presence of underlying medical issues, the procedure is likely to take longer.

When the procedure is over, you'll head to the recovery room and your eggs will head into the lab, whether off-site or within the same facility. While the embryology team is assessing your eggs, the medical team will continue to monitor your vital signs, ensure that you are not bleeding, and evaluate your pain, if any. Mild discomfort due to cramping and bloating is normal, but severe pain is not. Typically, within an hour the patient is snacking; drinking apple juice, coconut water, or ginger ale; taking a brief walk; and using the restroom, all of which are prerequisites for being released. The physician, whether it is your MD or the doctor on call, should then share the results with you. I meet with my patients before they leave to tell them the number of eggs we retrieved, and I remind them to take it easy as they recover from anesthesia.

The most difficult part of my job is telling a patient when a procedure is unsuccessful. Unfortunately, more than half of women who freeze their eggs at 37 years of age or older will find their efforts to be futile. It can be devastating for the patient and heart-wrenching for the provider as well. If there are far fewer than 70 percent that can be frozen, you should find out the cause and what can possibly be done to improve upon the results if you do another cycle.

Second to getting no eggs or no mature eggs at all, in my opinion, the biggest bummer of the process is not being able to assess the quality of the eggs extracted. It is impossible for your fertility doctor to tell you how many healthy versus unhealthy eggs have been frozen—no test, no visual clue, no assessment, no hints, no markers. Ten frozen eggs does not equal 10 babies. It could mean anywhere from zero to 10. When eggs are retrieved at a younger age and more are frozen, the odds that it could lead to a viable embryo at some point are increased, but there are no guarantees and no egg quality crystal ball that can make a prediction. The true value of egg freezing is only known when you thaw and fertilize eggs.

Post-op, the ovaries are still pretty swollen, so rigorous exercise is off limits, including jumping, twisting, sharp turning, running, or any activity that could impact your ovaries. (That includes sex.) The increased size of the ovaries puts them at risk for ovarian torsion, meaning no blood flow to the ovary, which can be a surgical emergency. It is a good idea to spend the rest of the day with your feet up, so most of my patients take the day off work. I also recommend eating something salty, like ramen, an everything bagel, or pizza, because salty foods help draw the fluid back into the blood vessels. Electrolyte-rich drinks will keep you hydrated and help with the fluid shifts that can occur after the retrieval. Increase your fiber because the high progesterone levels can lead to constipation, and add some protein to your diet to help with recovery. I tell my patients I will call them in the morning and always do. I hope yours does, too—you should never feel alone throughout the process.

After the procedure, there are typically no more shots, blood tests, or ultrasounds for that cycle. For five to 12 days following the extraction, you may still experience bloating, weight gain, fatigue, acne, or cramping. This is caused by the hormonal elevations and enlarged ovaries, but rest assured that it is temporary. Complications, both during and after the procedure, are rare. As someone who has overseen thousands of egg freezing cycles and connected with patients thoroughly about their experiences, I can tell you with confidence that the overall process is not as laborious or intrusive as some social media posts may lead you to believe. Some patients do report pain after the retrieval; every patient responds differently and has a different threshold for discomfort. Yes, you are poked and prodded in preparation for a retrieval, but it is absolutely false that you will need to miss weeks of work or significantly change your lifestyle. If needed, I recommend taking over-the-counter pain reliever for the first few days post-op, or I may need to prescribe a narcotic for some women with significantly high egg yields. You can continue to exercise, albeit in a modified fashion, enjoy your caffeine, and sip a cocktail.

Once the eggs are washed and analyzed, the embryologist will freeze only the eggs that are at the developmental stage appropriate for freezing. Remember the idea of synchronizing the eggs' race? We try to have them all win together, but they are not the Rockettes at the Christmas Spectacular, all kicking their legs in unison. There is almost always variability in a cohort of eggs, with some lagging behind (immature eggs) and others that are too ambitious (postmature eggs), but around 70 percent of them should be in sync and ripe for freezing. If more than 30 percent of the eggs are immature or postmature, this can suggest an underlying egg quality problem or issues with the egg stimulation medications, which would merit a conversation with your physician about any possible modifications should you undergo another cycle.

The mature eggs are frozen by being submerged in liquid nitrogen following the vitrification (fast-freeze) technique, going from fresh in a petri dish to frozen on a glass straw in less than 15 minutes. Two to three eggs are placed on each straw, which is about the diameter of a piece of spaghetti. They then make their way into a tank teeming with liquid nitrogen, whether at the clinic or at an on off-site storage facility, where they remain until you are ready to use them. In most clinics, each straw is labeled with the patient's name, date of birth, and unique identifier. All of the straws collectively are placed into a structure called a goblet, which is also labeled, and then placed into the tank.

Not everyone who freezes eggs decides to use them. Some people conceive naturally and do not need their eggs, while others may decide they do not want children. A large 2024 meta-analysis of 27 studies that encompassed 13,724 patients and over 17,000 egg freezing cycles found that only 10.8 percent of patients had returned to use their previously frozen eggs, and on average it took women seven years to return. We are still in the early days of large-scale egg freezing programs, and how many women ultimately return to use their eggs is largely unknown.

If you decide that you want to try to have a baby using your frozen eggs, whether it be with a partner or using donor sperm, it is recommended that you undergo genetic carrier testing to confirm that you and your sperm source do not overlap for any deleterious conditions. A blood or saliva sample can test for hundreds of conditions to reveal if you are a carrier for a myriad of recessive diseases. If an overlap is demonstrated, pregnancy is not off the table, but it may require further analysis and testing of an embryo before transfer. If no overlap is identified and all reproductive systems look good, you will get the green light from your fertility doctor to thaw eggs and try to fertilize them.

How many eggs you choose to thaw will depend on the number of eggs that were frozen, your age at the time of the freeze and thaw, and the family size you desire. For example, if you froze 15 eggs at age 28 and are now married and hoping to have two children with your partner, I would recommend thawing all of your eggs and fertilizing them with your partner's sperm. The extra embryo(s) that you don't transfer for your first child can remain frozen for your second or third child. In contrast, if you froze 20 eggs at age 24 and are currently 38 and single, looking to have a baby with donor sperm and hoping to maintain the ability to have a baby with a potential future partner, I would recommend only thawing a portion of your eggs. You don't want to put all of your "eggs in one basket"—yes, I use that line regularly—because you may want to keep some frozen for potential use with a partner. If you have a partner but want to maintain reproductive autonomy, I may suggest you don't touch your eggs at all. Instead, you may want to try to conceive with your eggs in vivo (inside the body) and leave the frozen eggs frozen should you need them down the road.

When you are ready, the embryology laboratory will schedule the egg thaw. Just as not all eggs are able to be frozen, not all eggs survive the thaw. Those that do survive the thaw, a statistic that is clinic dependent, will be injected with sperm. Given the hardness of previously frozen eggs' outer shell, it would be difficult for sperm to break through, so sperm is injected into the egg using a process called ICSI (intracytoplasmic sperm injection) in an attempt to achieve fertilization. About 18 hours later, the embryology team will check to see if the egg and sperm created any embryos. If they did, the embryos are monitored in the lab for a select number of days (usually between three and seven), and then are either transferred back into the uterus or are frozen for chromosomal analysis. In the latter situation, some clinics elect to grow embryos to the advanced stage, sample cells for chromosome screening, and freeze the embryo for possible future use, whether in months or years down the road. If the testing reveals the correct number of chromosomes, a transfer will occur in the subsequent menstrual cycle. I believe all embryos should undergo chromosomal screening, whether the eggs were previously frozen or extracted fresh. Without such data, if a pregnancy does not occur from the embryo transfer, a big piece of the "why did it not work?" question is missing. While some clinics caution patients against embryo freezing and chromosomal testing of embryos created from previously frozen eggs, high-quality embryology labs should feel confident in thawing eggs, biopsying and freezing the resultant embryos, and thawing them in the future.

Egg Freezing FAQs

How many eggs do I need to freeze to have a baby?
While there are online fertility calculators that offer estimates based on your age, there is no magic number that is a surefire answer. We do know that the

more you have, the better, and that the younger you freeze the eggs, the more potential they will have. Decisions on how many eggs to freeze must be made on an individual basis with your doctor, who knows your fertility history and what you hope your fertility future will look like.

Will you know if my eggs are good?
Currently, there is no test that can shed light on the quality of eggs or their ability to make a baby. Sure, as an experienced clinician there are red flags during an egg freezing cycle that give me pause, but data on egg potential is not available until the eggs are thawed, fertilized by a sperm, grown in the laboratory, and transferred back into the uterus. However, the younger you freeze and the more eggs you get, the better your chances of success down the road.

If I freeze my eggs, does that push me closer to menopause faster?
Nope. Whether you freeze eggs or not, they will die off after that menstrual cycle is over (the medical term for this is *atresia*). Simply stated, if you do not use them, you lose them. Undergoing an egg freezing procedure will not speed up the pace of egg loss.

If I freeze my eggs, do they degrade over time?
Eggs (and embryos) are not like chicken in the freezer that should be trashed once covered in ice crystals after a year or two. Once the eggs are submerged in liquid nitrogen, they can remain frozen indefinitely, with no decline in their quality. There are no laws in the United States dictating how long they can be frozen, but the ASRM does not encourage carrying a pregnancy after age 55. If pregnancy is still desired, gestational surrogacy can be considered.

What can I do to improve my egg quality?
While there is some data supporting the use of supplements, dietary changes, acupuncture, and lifestyle modifications, none have been definitively proven to improve egg quality. We cannot change what we have or reverse the aging clock.

If I freeze my eggs, will that prevent my ability to get pregnant naturally?
Absolutely not! The eggs we freeze during a round of egg freezing would have been lost if you did not freeze them, so you are not pushing yourself closer to menopause or hurting your chances of getting pregnant. We know this not only from those who have frozen eggs but also from women who donate their eggs. Women can donate their eggs time and time again without any negative impact on their fertility.

Do I have to stop the pill to do egg freezing?
Yes, you must stop your oral contraceptive pill before initiating an egg freezing cycle. The pill is like Ambien for your ovaries. It puts them to sleep. We need them to be awake to respond to fertility medication. Ideally we recommend that women stop their pill at least one month before starting their fertility medications.

Do I have to remove an IUD to do egg freezing?
An IUD, whether hormonal or nonhormonal, does not need to be removed before starting an egg freezing cycle. Even without periods, blood work can guide us on when is the ideal time to start the medications. Additionally, the presence of the IUD does not decrease the success rates of the egg freezing cycle.

Do I have to change what I eat, drink, or do in the gym if I undergo egg freezing?
Most activities do not need to be modified when going through the egg freezing process. There is no diet that will change the cycle outcome, nor is there any amount of alcohol that will impact egg quality. While I do not recommend McDonald's and a bottle of wine on the daily, cutting out gluten, dairy, and alcohol is most certainly not going to impact your egg freezing cycle. When it comes to exercise, you do need to make modifications; jumping, running, twisting, and turning should be limited both during and immediately after the procedure. This is not because activity will impact egg quality but because it can increase the risk of an ovary twisting (medical term: torsion), which is a surgical emergency.

Can I have heterosexual sex while taking the shots?
This is a no, absolutely not, and it is a very bad idea. Having heterosexual intercourse during the stimulation process can result in an undesired pregnancy. Even the best fertility doctors can unintentionally leave an egg behind during the egg retrieval. Sperm + egg = possible pregnancy, but knock yourself out with other forms of pleasure. In general, nothing inside the vagina is advised, as ovaries can get to be five times their normal size and could become impacted. As such, intercourse is likely to be unpleasurable.

Ice, Ice Baby

I think of egg and embryo freezing as two sports games that follow the same playbook for the first half, then significantly diverge after the halftime show. With embryo freezing, your eggs do not hit the freezer solo because they first get fertilized by sperm.

After eggs are extracted from the ovaries and prepped by the embryologist, they get ready to meet their mates (a.k.a. sperm). Fertilization can be achieved in two ways: insemination or ICSI. In "insem" cases, most labs will place approximately 50,000 sperm in a drop of media that contains two to four eggs. The number of sperm will vary based on the sample as a more concentrated sperm sample, needs fewer sperm in the drop. Ultimately, the hope is that one will penetrate the outside of the egg and achieve fertilization. It only takes one! Fertilization occurs outside of the body but in very much the same way that it would inside the body, with thousands of sperm vying for the gold, if you will, and one claiming the title with fertilization. With ICSI, on the other hand, an embryologist will select one sperm and inject it into the egg. This method is frequently used in cases with poor sperm quantity or quality, a history of poor fertilization, or when accurate genetic testing of the embryo is a high priority.

It takes around 16 to 20 hours for an embryologist to determine how many of the egg and sperm combinations have become embryos. The presence of two pronuclei, one from the sperm and one from the egg, is the marker of successful fertilization and early embryo development. The pronuclei of the sperm and egg should contain 23 chromosomes, half of the total genetic material needed to make a healthy embryo with 46 chromosomes. Older eggs are more likely to be released with too many or too few chromosomes, leading to abnormal embryos. Over a period of five to seven days, the embryos are nurtured in a laboratory with specific parameters, such as ambient air quality conditions and the secret sauce that the embryos grow in, called the culture media. All these variables promote development, from a two-cell embryo to a more advanced embryo called a blastocyst. Embryos that cannot survive in a high-quality embryology lab cannot make it in the body either, so in some ways it is like undergoing natural selection, albeit in an unnatural fashion. Extended embryo culture, the practice of growing embryos past the cleavage (day three) stage, helps identify the highest quality embryos, which are most likely to carry the correct number of chromosomes. To enhance analysis, embryologists can also take cells from the trophectoderm, which will hopefully become the placenta, for further biopsy and analysis. A by-product of knowing an embryo's chromosome number is the ability to identify an embryo's gender. The X and Y chromosomes are analyzed during the process and, if the couple desires, can be shared. While some couples will come and make embryos solely to know the gender, sex selection is not a routine practice.

Immediately following the biopsy procedure but before results are back, embryos are frozen. Remember, unlike that chicken in the freezer, once embryos hit the liquid nitrogen, there is not an expiration date, nor do they degrade over time. Many large-scale studies have demonstrated no impact of prolonged freezing on embryo survival, clinical pregnancy, implantation, miscarriage, and live birth. It takes approximately two to three weeks for genetic testing results to identify which embryos harbor the correct number of chromosomes and what the options are for next steps. The testing, combined with information obtained in the embryology lab, has evolved significantly so that we can determine not only if an embryo has the correct number of chromosomes but also which are more likely to transfer successfully and result in a live birth. The testing also ensures that, when present in the gamete sources, single-gene recessive conditions, like CF, or dominant conditions, such as the BRCA gene, are not passed down to the next generation. The advent of large-scale and rapid sequencing, called expanded carrier screening (ECS), has made it possible to screen for many conditions in a single blood test before starting the embryo freezing process, allowing for more testing of embryos for single gene mutations down the road.

Time for another sports analogy: After embryos are tasked with surviving in the lab and undergoing genetic testing, you may only have a few players left on the field or just one last man (or woman!) standing. Whether it is one or a few, these embryos are your MVPs. In high-quality labs, advanced embryos with the correct number of chromosomes now can translate into live birth rates 50 to 70 percent of the time. By proving that they can make it to the championship game, if you will, they have shown they are tough, resilient, and ready for the road ahead. In general, I recommend that couples have around two healthy embryos for every one child they hope to have. At a hit rate of 50 to 70 percent, that should cover the odds. This stat assumes that the intrauterine environment is hospitable; for those with known or suspected uterine pathology, more embryos may be required.

When you decide it is time to start or add to your family, you can head to your bullpen, a.k.a. the clinic, and call up your closer, a.k.a. a frozen embryo (typically only one at a time, but that can vary). After an evaluation by your fertility doctor confirming no contraindications to pregnancy, a healthy uterus, and other preimplantation considerations, the transfer process can commence. In the three weeks leading up to the transfer, a handful of medications combined with a few blood tests and ultrasounds will ensure that the uterus is ready for the main event. With the help of a team that may include a nurse, embryologist and physician, the embryo makes its way from the lab into your uterus through a process that is no more rigorous than a pap smear. While no one loves a speculum, you don't have to worry about much else. If you have a partner, they are typically invited to the transfer party, which is a painless and quick event. Bed rest is not required, and you can resume your normal activities. Nine days later, a blood test will reveal if the embryo implanted successfully in your uterus.

Embryo Disposition

What happens if you do not want to use any or all of the embryos you had frozen? This is something you need to think about when you begin the process, not on the tail end. Decisions regarding embryo disposition are made before embryos are created. If you have ever had a medical procedure in which you have been handed a bunch of forms to sign and you barely read a word of it before scribbling your signature, I get it. It seems like a bunch of irrelevant consent forms and gibberish, so you just initial it straight down the line. I urge you not to do that in this case. This is different. You must not only read the fine print when a clinic presents you with consent forms but also give it a lot of thought.

Embryos, like any marital or partnered asset, are joint property of both individuals who created the embryos. Think of embryo freezing as a marriage, one that must have a prenup of sorts. In this case it is called a disposition agreement, and the consequences without one can be disastrous. Deciding what to do with the embryos as a harmonious couple can be challenging, so imagine how the scene will turn if the relationship ends. I recommend meeting with a reproductive lawyer (yes, that's a thing) to make sure you and your sperm source are crystal clear on what will happen with any unused embryos and to help sort through any legal and emotional issues connected to embryo disposition. Scenarios that are accounted for in a disposition agreement include the death of self (the female partner whose eggs are extracted); death of the partner; simultaneous death; dissolution of the relationship; and age-limiting factors, meaning what happens to the embryos after each partner reaches a certain age or a combined age. For each of these events, couples and individuals typically discard embryos, donate embryos to research, or defer to a court decree. Sometimes couples opt to donate embryos to another couple, which requires legal counsel and an addendum to the consent. This is frequently referred to as embryo donation or embryo adoption. While the terms are used interchangeably, adoption refers to living children whereas embryo donation is a medical procedure. This is done infrequently and largely driven by faith-based organizations, but there are some clinics that offer it without religious restrictions. In some cases, albeit less frequently, couples may elect for a "compassionate transfer" as a means of disposition. This entails placing an embryo back in the uterus at an inopportune time, knowing the uterus cannot accept it, so it will not lead to a viable pregnancy, thereby avoiding the need to discard or donate them.

When sperm or eggs are donated anonymously, rights are waived, so the donor has no leverage to tell you what to do or not do with their gametes. There is no need to contact the donor source when making decisions about any unused embryos containing their tissue. If the source of sperm or eggs was a directed donor, then there is a contract signed at the time of securing the gamete indicating what you can or cannot do with any embryos containing their DNA.

Back to my daughters' questions about who I like better, the answer when it comes to them and to frozen gametes is still a resounding "Both!"

I often ask patients who need help deciding which course of action to pursue: "Do you want data in real time, or are you comfortable knowing that potential for pregnancy exists along with the option for a future sperm source of your choosing?" The fact that we even have options like egg or embryo freezing, both with excellent success rates, is astounding. We are fortunate to have effective ways to sidestep the limits of our ovaries. There is no one right answer, but there is the life-changing possibility of shaping your reproductive future.

PART 2

SOLVING THE INFERTILITY PUZZLE

CHAPTER 5

When Conceiving Isn't Easy

As I've said throughout this book, women become infertile as we age. Before we take our first breath outside of the womb, we are on the road to diminished egg quantity and quality, a one-way street that leads to a dead end before we may expect it. (A man's fertility declines with age, too, but a woman's runway is much shorter.) The relatively new field of fertility preservation offers choices that can circumvent this inevitable outcome and various work-arounds that have transformed reproduction. But what if you are already struggling with infertility, or in the future you experience difficulty getting pregnant? Whether you are early in the process, deep in the trenches of disappointment after disappointment, or thinking about possible challenges down the road, my aim is to help you navigate infertility with clarity and competence. This chapter unravels causes of and treatments for infertility, many of which have evolved in recent years.

The WHO reports that one in six individuals suffers from infertility, meaning 50 million couples or 186 million individuals have difficulty conceiving. Much to everyone's despair, asking Google or ChatGPT: "What could be making me infertile and how can I treat it?" will get you no usable answers. Infertility is a complex medical disease that requires years of training and clinical practice to identify, diagnose, and treat. In the "olden" days—meaning a couple of years ago—infertility was defined as the inability to get pregnant after six months to a year of unprotected sex, depending on one's age. In Part 1, I touched on how the changing definition of infertility impacts fertility preservation, but it has even more significant repercussions for infertility treatment.

According to the prior definition, heterosexual couples with a woman under age 35 would need to have unprotected sex for a year before they could be diagnosed as infertile. Women over 35 could be diagnosed with infertility after six months of trying to conceive since the odds of conceiving are reduced with age. Only after a diagnosis six months to one year later could treatment possibly be covered by insurance if infertility benefits were available. What a waste of precious time for a woman who is 34 with a risk factor for infertility, like a mom with early menopause, to keep trying for an entire year before uncovering and then hopefully addressing any underlying issues or the likely root of the problem, which is often age. Imagine a 40-year-old in perimenopause who finds the love of her life and wants to start a family right away, only to be told she needs to try conceiving for six months before accessing treatment. Time is not on her side, so waiting six months could be the difference between having a genetic child versus needing to use a donor egg. Either can be an excellent option, but these are choices we should not be making based on limiting, outdated definitions.

How about a woman who wants to become a single parent by choice? Based on the old definition, with whom was she to be having unprotected sex before insurance might have deemed her eligible for medical intervention? Likewise, for same-sex couples the burden to prove infertility was discriminatory and often detrimental, as access to suitable care was limited for much of the patient population.

These are not just theoretical scenarios. I have ridden the merry-go-round of frustration and despair with so many patients, one of whom is in the midst of a class-action lawsuit against an insurance provider. My patient and her wife, who wanted to have a baby, had two sets of ovaries and two uteri, but no sperm—so clearly they would need to procure sperm and proceed with medical intervention to build a family. Although they had expansive fertility benefits, insurance refused to cover several rounds of intrauterine insemination (IUI) with donor sperm because they had not been trying to conceive for a year, in accordance with the definition of infertility at that time. My patient, who is now the mom to both a little girl and boy thanks to IVF, was forced to pay out of pocket. She is now hoping to recoup some of that cost as well as ensure that others have access to reproductive care without discrimination based on gender, sexuality, or any other factors. Other similar lawsuits have recently been filed by people claiming their access to reproductive care was unfairly compromised, so my patient's case may be precedent setting.

Which brings us to the updated definition of infertility, a groundbreaking step forward when, in 2023, the ASRM redefined infertility as a disease or condition characterized by the inability to get pregnant because of the patient's medical, sexual and reproductive history, age, physical findings and diagnostic testing, as well as the need for donor eggs or sperm to achieve pregnancy. The ASRM explicitly states, "Nothing in this definition shall be used to deny or delay treatment to any individual, regardless of relationship status or sexual orientation." Drop the mic! It is a game-changer for anyone who needs help conceiving—gay or straight, male or female, single or partnered, in their 20s or in their 40s, suffering from early menopause or fertile as can be—to be able to access reproductive treatment. Infertility is not straightforward and family-building can take many forms, so this more inclusive definition ensures that parenting is not a club with VIP privileges for some.

The definition of infertility may be new, but the existence of infertility dates back to ancient times. Medical texts in ancient Egypt and Greece touch on infertility, and early in the Old Testament, Sarah and Abraham struggle to conceive a child. Three of the four matriarchs in the Judeo-Christian tradition are deemed barren as well as many others in the Bible, so clearly it is a noteworthy narrative. Until the mid- to late 1800s, those who struggled with infertility might consider prayer, fasting, chanting spells, or going on a pilgrimage as an antidote to childlessness, which was perceived as a punishment from God. Some doctors believed infertility was a psychosomatic condition and suggested adoption to alleviate a woman's disappointment, stress, or obsessiveness, after which point a pregnancy would be more likely.

Since the beginning of time, infertility carried a social stigma and left women struggling in shame, guilt, and fear. From ancient Egypt to medieval Japan to 16th-century England, examples abound of women whose inability to bear children led to divorce, discrimination, and disgrace. They were ostracized from their communities, blamed, deemed less valuable, and left to suffer in silence. With a woman's value predicated on being able to bear children, marriage agreements were not completed until after childbirth, and a major cause of divorce was what was thought to be a woman's struggle to conceive. We now know that male contribution to infertility is significant, but for hundreds of years it was viewed solely as a female problem.

For much of the early 1800s, medical solutions for infertility were dominated by gynecological surgical procedures, which led to complications and had limited success rates. Not until the 20th century did IUI become reliably successful, once scientists discovered the need to wash sperm before placing the fastest swimmers into the uterus at the optimal time, giving them a head start by bypassing the vagina and the cervix. By the 1930s, the role of estrogen and progesterone in human reproduction was identified, and synthetic versions of these hormones were developed in the 1940s. In the 1970s, scientists identified the hormones that are essential for ovarian stimulation: FSH and LH. Initially, they were extracted from the urine of menopausal women (crazy, right?) to help younger women who needed a boost of these hormones. Ultimately, their ability to be produced in a laboratory and administered, at first intramuscularly and then subcutaneously, would transform fertility treatment by triggering the production of multiple eggs.

IVF was another huge development in the field. Conceiving life outside the body began when Gregory Pincus, who is best known for his coinvention of the birth control pill, experimented successfully with IVF in rabbits in the 1930s, proving that it was possible. More than a decade later, in 1944, it was the work of Miriam Menkin, a lab technician in Massachusetts, that resulted in the first fertilization of egg and sperm outside the body. Incidentally, Menkin had been denied entry into medical school, as most women were at the time, and her nickname was the "egg chaser" because her job entailed running ovarian tissue from the operating room to the lab where she worked three flights up.

There are many other pioneers who paved the way for the modern-day practice of IVF, some of whom were covered previously. Most notably were Patrick Steptoe and Robert Edwards, whose work led to the 1978 birth of the world's first IVF baby, colloquially referred to as the first test-tube baby, Louise Brown. In 1980, the first IVF clinic was opened in the United States by Drs. Georgeanna and Howard Jones. The following year, it was in their clinic in Norfolk, Virginia, that the first American IVF baby, Elizabeth Carr, was born.

In the early days of IVF, women were hospitalized for invasive abdominal surgeries to extract frequently immature eggs, as physicians essentially guessed (albeit educated guesses based on the limited data they were working with) at the best timing for surgery to extract eggs by collecting buckets of urine to identify elevations in hormones. Multiple embryos were placed back into fallopian tubes rather than into the uterus, and success rates were poor. By the mid-1980s, ovarian stimulation fueled the production of multiple eggs. Moving from a natural cycle to a stimulated cycle, along with optimizing the timing of retrieval and adding medications to prevent premature ovulation, allowed physicians to increase egg yield, which drastically increased the odds of getting pregnant.

Other developments included tracking follicular development with blood tests to measure hormone levels, and vaginal ultrasound measurements to track follicle size. Labs also transformed IVF by identifying the essential ingredients needed in the culture media in which to grow an embryo, extending embryo culture, performing embryo biopsy, and improving genetic analysis platforms. In short, over the course of around 50 years, treatment for infertility, including IVF, became significantly more dependable, with high success rates measured not only by achieving a pregnancy but also by having a healthy child. We *have* come a long way, baby.

As astounding as the medical advancements that led to IVF are, they were not accessible to all of the people who needed them for far too long. Infertility was not recognized as a medical disease by the WHO until 2009, and another eight years passed before the American Medical Association (AMA) did the same. Without this distinction, insurance coverage was limited and access to care restrictive, leaving countless people to suffer physically, emotionally, and financially.

One in five people worldwide will develop cancer, a number not dissimilar to the one in six who suffer from infertility. I make that comparison to drive home how common infertility is, and also to contrast how differently we view the disease of cancer versus the disease of infertility. Cancer patients seeking care are not told to suffer in silence or to relax until the desired outcome arrives when it is meant to. Similarly, those suffering from infertility deserve access to treatment, not condescending and medically inaccurate platitudes, or even worse, explicit denial of care. It is long overdue, but thankfully, the approximately 18 percent of the population who suffer from infertility increasingly have safe, effective, and increasingly affordable options for medical treatment.

No longer do women, men, or couples need to seek unproven remedies, resort to self-blame, or be denied coverage for treating the medical disease of infertility. The field of reproductive medicine—and a society that has slowly but surely embraced the remarkable advancements—has changed how women can get pregnant, how families are formed, when childbearing can occur, and so much more. Success rates have soared from single digits per IVF cycle to close to 80 percent per embryo transfer in select centers and cases. Not only has insurance coverage for infertility increased, but 11 states, at this time, have mandated both IVF and fertility preservation coverage, and an additional two states have mandated only IVF coverage.

Today it is estimated that every 15 seconds a batch of human eggs is extracted from a woman somewhere on this planet. Every 15 seconds! Since the 1978 birth of the first test-tube baby, Louise Brown, it is estimated that more than 13 million babies worldwide have been born using ART. In 2023, there were 95,860 babies born in the United States using ART, and around 2.5 percent of all babies born in the United States are the result of ART. Worldwide, that number is estimated to be 500,000 babies each year. In certain European countries, like Denmark, Spain, and Greece, ART births make up 8 to 10 percent of all births, a statistic that continues to grow as infertility rises due to a confluence of factors, with people waiting longer to conceive at the top of the list.

As infertility rates rise, economists, population experts, and governments are preparing for a global problem when the fertility replacement rate drops below the number needed to maintain the population. By 2050, over three-quarters of countries will not have high enough fertility rates to sustain their populations, and by 2100 it is estimated that will apply to 97 percent of countries. Such declines are, in part, impacted by people choosing to remain childless, which is a valid decision in its own right, but the rise in fertility struggles has also contributed significantly to the emerging threat of underpopulation. Recognizing the negative impact that dipping below the replacement level can have on the prosperity and security of a nation, some countries, like Japan and South Korea, offer government-subsidized ART treatment to fuel procreation.

If the sheer number of babies born via IVF or other forms of ART doesn't provide enough proof of infertility as a common disease accompanied by a growing need for intervention, following the money sure does. Thousands of fertility clinics have opened across the globe, supporting people who struggle with infertility or need medical intervention to build a family. The US market for fertility clinic services, including revenue generated by fertility clinics providing treatments like IVF, egg freezing, embryo freezing, and IUI, was estimated at $7.9 billion in 2022 and is forecast to grow at a rate of roughly 13.5 percent annually to reach $16.8 billion by the end of 2028. The global fertility services market size, a value that encompasses treatments, medications, and diagnostics, is expected to increase from approximately $45 billion in 2025 to $92 billion in 2033. While some of this growth can be attributed to fertility preservation as a growing subset of the field, a newfound focus on helping all patients who suffer from infertility is also a huge factor.

In recent years, the veil of shame and secrecy associated with infertility has begun to lift, allowing a growing number of people to finally seek treatment without prejudice, discrimination, or bearing the brunt of social stigma. In my own waiting room, not too long ago people sat with their heads down until their name was called, then surreptitiously went behind closed doors and spoke in hushed tones about their failed efforts to get pregnant. Now, while my waiting room is not exactly as social as cocktail hour, the aura of embarrassment or discomfort has dissipated substantially. Patients make referrals to their friends not all that differently than if they were recommending a plumber, and even document their journeys on social media.

Celebrities have also helped normalize the struggle to conceive by sharing their stories. From Chrissy Teigen and John Legend's multiple IVF cycles and surrogacy to Kourtney Kardashian and Travis Barker's failed IVF cycles before conceiving naturally, public figures have helped illuminate for women and couples that building a family is not necessarily straightforward. Other celebrities whose challenges conceiving have helped raise awareness about infertility include Courteney Cox, Gabrielle Union, Brooke Shields, Nicole Kidman, Celine Dion, Khloé Kardashian, and Tyra Banks. National Infertility Awareness Week has made inroads with prominent ad campaigns, and World IVF Day, which recognizes advances in fertility medicine since Louise Brown's birth, continues to raise awareness and advocacy.

The prevalence of infertility and the utilization of IVF or other medical interventions to build a family drew unprecedented attention during the 2024 presidential campaign, when former First Lady Michelle Obama, vice presidential candidate Tim Walz, and Senator Tammy Duckworth each shared their family's struggles. This candor on the campaign trail may have been politically motivated, as reproductive rights have become a polarizing issue, but the need for people to build families in all kinds of ways crosses party lines. Whether you are a Democrat or a Republican, live in a state that protects reproductive rights or challenges them, are beginning or ending a journey with infertility, the data is clear that infertility is a common disease and that modern medicine is successful in treating it.

Patient POV

Sabrina, 39

We were two women in our 30s who decided to start a family during the pandemic while much of the world was still working from home. After we both got checked out, the doctor advised that I was better positioned to do the egg retrieval and carry. Our first retrieval using donor sperm led to no viable embryos, which was pretty upsetting. As a high achiever with no fertility issues, I definitely did not think we would come up empty-handed. The quality of eggs that round wasn't our best, I was told, which can happen sometimes. Our doctor changed the treatment regimen, including switching up some of the medications, and in the next round we got three viable, high-quality embryos: two girls and a boy. During the transfer, it was wild to see the two little embryos on the screen get shot into my uterus. Only one took, and that embryo became our now three-year-old daughter, Willow.

Given that we only had one embryo left, we decided to do another round of IVF. I stopped breastfeeding, got my period, and went straight into the round. We were away for a long weekend when I realized I forgot one of the drugs, which meant we had to make some modifications to the plan. It was pretty irresponsible of me, but maybe my head was so consumed with mixing needles like a chemist and then injecting myself while in a bathroom stall at a restaurant or in my car parked at the beach. The things we do for our families, even while we're building them! All's well that ends well because we got two healthy girl embryos.

We did our second transfer when Willow was eight months old and brought her with us. I think it was a first for the doctor and embryologist to have a baby accompany the patient in the procedure room! Nine days later, we found out I was pregnant with our second daughter, whom we named Penelope. Maybe it's easy for me to say this given our successful outcome, but my advice to other women is to stay positive. Also, we loved our clinic so much that they became like my family. Every day I still feel overwhelming gratitude, including that I was lucky enough to have insurance coverage. My girls are my world.

Causes of Infertility

A puzzle is my go-to metaphor to explain infertility. This puzzle has five primary pieces: two for the ovaries (one for ovulation and another for egg quantity and quality); one for fallopian tubes; one for uterus; and one for sperm. A female patient needs to release an egg through ovulation, at least one fallopian tube needs to be open, the uterus needs to be able to accept an embryo, and the male partner has to have healthy sperm that can swim and fertilize an egg. There are numerous aspects of infertility within each of those big pieces, along with a mystery piece for when causes of infertility cannot be pinpointed, but those five are the basics.

When a patient or couple comes in after unsuccessfully trying to get pregnant, it is my job to uncover where and why the pieces are not coming together. I think of myself as a detective charged with figuring out which missing piece will make the puzzle whole, leading to a healthy pregnancy. Remember the board game Clue? We'd try to solve the mystery by guessing something like "Professor Plum in the conservatory with a candlestick." Unlike the board game, my tools are diagnostic tests, my experience, and my patients' health history, and then I'm charged with speculating who, or more accurately what, the culprit could be. If I see that both fallopian tubes are open, then I am likely to make my way toward the ovaries and uterus. If one partner looks all clear, then the other is my next suspect. Despite all the advances in fertility treatment, diagnostics for infertility can be limited. There is still no way to evaluate egg quality, researchers are still in the dark about why some uteri cannot accept healthy embryos, nor can a semen analysis reveal if a sperm has the ability to fertilize an egg. But that does not mean that Professor Plum loses the game. I just have to work harder to analyze each piece of the puzzle to figure out why they aren't fitting just right.

If that metaphor does not speak to you, then imagine a factory assembly line. Whether the visual you see is the OG Ford Model T car; Lucy and Ethel at the chocolate factory; or a more modern-day, automated, robotic bottling of beverages, the themes of efficiency, productivity, and volume come into focus. If one part of the assembly line decides to take a break or stop following instructions, the whole process comes to a halt. Until that one part is back in the game, overall output remains at a standstill. All hands must be on deck, or there is no production and no product. Likewise, infertility is what happens when the reproductive factory lines, on either the male or female sides, or both, are interrupted. When any one part stops doing their job or does it inefficiently—whether that's ovulation, egg quantity/quality, fallopian tubes, uterus, sperm, brain, thyroid, or any of the other workers on the line—the output of a fertile individual or couple becomes one that is struggling to conceive or deemed infertile.

About 30 percent of infertility cases are attributed solely to the female partner, 30 percent solely to the male partner, 20 percent to a combination of both, and 20 percent of cases are unexplained. About a quarter of the time, there are multiple factors contributing to infertility. These percentages can fluctuate, with factors like geography playing a role. In major metropolitan cities, where couples may start families at a later age than in rural areas, there is likely to be more female age-related infertility. (Eggs age. Heard me say that before?) The exact percentages may vary, but the gist is the same: Infertility can be the result of both sperm and egg source. For a woman, causes of infertility may include poor egg quality or quantity, blockage of the fallopian tubes, or an ovarian disorder. For a man, infertility may be caused by an inability to produce sperm, abnormal sperm, sperm that can't swim, or blockage in the ejection of semen. There are also countless cases of unexplained infertility, meaning no cause can be identified, or if a cause exists, it cannot be measured or tested.

Someone struggling to conceive may not want to be bothered with what can seem like semantics, but the difference between primary infertility and secondary infertility is really important. Primary infertility describes a couple or an individual that has never conceived a pregnancy of any kind, including a biochemical pregnancy (in which pregnancy hormone is detected in the blood or urine but not on ultrasound), a pregnancy that resulted in a miscarriage, or a termination. Secondary infertility describes a couple or individual that has conceived a pregnancy in the past but not necessarily a healthy one. (There are nuances to this definition, but that is a simplistic way of explaining the gist.) The distinction between the two can shed light on what may be causing the problem and how best to treat it. Primary infertility is slightly less common and, at least for me, usually more challenging to solve, especially in couples under 35 who have been having regular intercourse. The diagnosis can be more complicated to uncover, and the traditional treatments, including oral medications, IUI, and IVF, can be hit or miss since we do not always know the exact source of the issue. Secondary infertility is slightly more common, and its most frequent cause is the decline of egg quantity and quality as a result of female age. If, for example, a patient conceived her first child at 33, and then tries unsuccessfully for a second child at 36, I am less likely to be scratching my head as to why. Having one kind of infertility does not mean you won't also be inflicted by the other kind at some point, as some people may be diagnosed with uterine infertility and subsequently struggle to conceive due to ovulatory dysfunction. Conversely, you are not at higher risk for a second type of infertility by virtue of having a prior diagnosis. Couples that need treatment to conceive their first child, for example, are often shocked when their second comes along by surprise, so rest assured that infertility is often both treatable and fluid.

Patient POV

Izzy, 46

My husband and I have been together since high school, and we always shared the dream of having a large family. Over the course of trying to make that dream a reality, I experienced eight miscarriages, a bout of toxoplasmosis early during my pregnancy with our first child, and the need for debilitating immunotherapy treatments. Although I did eventually manage to safely deliver two full-term babies, it was clear that my body did not like pregnancy. After two more miscarriages when we started trying for our third child, we decided that enough was enough. My body and mind were maxed out. I felt that I was not doing my marriage or my two healthy, young children any favors by staying on the fertility roller coaster.

My husband and I decided that gestational surrogacy was a path we wanted to explore. At the time, gestational surrogacy was not legal in our state, so we chose an out-of-state doctor and agency, and got matched with a thoroughly vetted, experienced carrier who lived in Ohio, a surrogacy-friendly state. The medical process on my end was as straightforward as a round of IVF, but with an extra layer of FDA testing added to the embryo so that it could be legally implanted in another woman's uterus.

I got to know and trust our surrogate over the phone before meeting her in person on transfer day. I had a few frustrations over the course of her pregnancy, but reminded myself that she was doing her best, which was better than

I could do. I treated her like a true partner, thinking that the more respect I gave her, the more love she would have for the baby she was growing. When our baby was born, my husband and I were in the delivery room along with our surrogate's mother and husband. I got a hospital room next door to the surrogate for two nights and gave the surrogate full access to the baby in the nursery. As far as I was concerned, she had carried him for nine months and had a bond with him, so I wanted to give her whatever she needed to bring her experience full circle.

I always say that my third baby was "my best pregnancy." I thought about the pregnancy every single day, but having a bit of separation from the process after so many years of traumatic reproductive experiences was really healthy for me. I felt emotionally lighter, was finally able to give my two toddlers the focus they deserved, and wasn't suffering through months of grueling medical treatments. I didn't feel like any less of a mom for not carrying that pregnancy. I knew it was the right choice and actually wished I'd saved myself years of anguish by turning to surrogacy earlier. Surrogacy, it turns out, is really a story of enormous love, determination, and sacrifice on the part of so many people, one that we've always wanted our son to feel good about. He knows that we wanted him so badly that we did everything we could to bring him into this world.

The list of causes for both primary and secondary infertility is long, with plenty of overlap because the puzzle pieces of infertility are not always clear-cut. These are some of the most common causes of infertility, with brief explanations to help you understand the basics of treatment.

OVULATORY DYSFUNCTION: Every 21 to 35 days, the big event in the menstrual cycle occurs for most women when an egg is released from the ovary. This is ovulation, which happens smack in the middle of the menstrual cycle's two phases, the follicular phase and the luteal phase. Ovulation sets the cadence and regularity of the menstrual cycle, so when a period is abnormal, irregular, or nonexistent, that is the hallmark of ovulatory dysfunction. (If you studied Latin, you might appreciate that complete cessation of ovulation is called anovulation and irregular ovulation is called oligoovulation.)

Most women have two ovaries. Ovulation does not necessarily follow a consistent left, right, left, right pattern, but it does alternate between the two ovaries. Think of a football team executing a play as they march down the field toward the end zone. That is the follicular phase, around nine to 20 days, which is focused on growing the follicle and developing the egg. When the end zone is in sight, ovulation occurs. The brain, specifically the hypothalamus, must send signals to the pituitary, and in turn to the ovaries, one of which ultimately throws the final pass into the end zone. That final throw before the ball flies through the air into the end zone is ovulation, the release of an egg. Ovulation occurs earlier in women with shorter cycles and later in women with longer cycles. If any of the players are not in sync, somebody fumbles the ball, or the quarterback gets sacked, then the ball—in this case, the egg—does not make it down the field or out of the ovary. The luteal phase focuses on the hormones needed should a pregnancy occur, including developing what's called a corpus luteum, a mass of cells. If there is no developing follicle, there will be no egg released, no ovulation, no corpus luteum, and then it is pretty clear that ovulatory dysfunction is at play. Alternatively, there could be plenty of eggs and follicles, but if the signals are not coming out in a systematic fashion, the playbook is in disarray. In the case with PCOS, for example, no ovulation will occur.

The code crackers to diagnose underlying ovulation issues include a blood test to measure progesterone levels, ultrasound to look for the presence of a corpus luteum, urine ovulation prediction kit to look for a rise of LH in urine, or a basal body temperature shift, as an elevation can indicate ovulation. Causes of ovulatory dysfunction can result from both reproductive and nonreproductive organs. They include hypothalamic dysfunction, thyroid disorders, hyperprolactinemia, PCOS, early menopause/ovarian failure, congenital adrenal hyperplasia, extreme weight loss/weight gain, diabetes, autoimmune diseases, excessive stress or exercise, and select medications. Treatment can include oral medications or injectable hormones designed to reinstate ovulation, depending on the exact source of the dysfunction. If a patient, for example, is too thin, overexercises, is overweight, or has PCOS, then modifying lifestyle may also be advised before turning to medications.

DIMINISHED OVARIAN RESERVE: Just as my daughters are sick of me yelling at them to hang up their wet towels, you are probably getting tired of hearing this, but that won't stop me from saying it again: A woman's egg supply is limited and likely to tap out before we want. As women wait to have children, coupled with our longer modern-day lifespan, the runway we have is seemingly getting shorter and shorter. As such, diminished egg quantity or quality, medically termed diminished ovarian reserve (DOR), is a very common cause of infertility, particularly in women older than 35. Advanced age is the most common cause of DOR, but other culprits include ovarian surgery, pelvic radiation, certain chemotherapeutic agents, genetic mutations, endometriosis, and medications that can cause diminished ovarian reserve.

A diagnosis of DOR in an individual or couple struggling with infertility is typically made either by measuring the antral follicle count (AFC) on ultrasound or by analyzing hormone levels (FSH, AMH) in the blood. Treatments are usually focused on achieving superovulation (ovulating more than one egg) to increase the chances of releasing a healthy egg, either with oral medications or injectable hormones followed by IUI or IVF.

TUBAL DISEASE: The tubes are the tunnels that connect the ovaries to the uterus, and most women have two of them. After an egg is ovulated from the ovary, it is picked up by the adjacent fallopian tube, where it hangs out until it meets up with a sperm or disintegrates. Once sperm enters the female reproductive tract through the vagina, makes its way through the cervix, into the uterus and then the tubes, fertilization can occur if the sperm and egg happen to bump into each other. Like star-crossed lovers with a ticking clock soundtrack, that meetup is no small feat and happens faster than the average American woman can run a 5K. (If you're curious, that's 41 minutes and 21 seconds.)

As anyone who has been to New York City or New Jersey can attest, a blocked tunnel makes exiting or entering the city from New Jersey, Brooklyn, or Queens an absolute nightmare. Traffic comes to a standstill while horns start honking and angry drivers shout expletives. Likewise, when one or more fallopian tubes are blocked, nothing can get through, not even the teeny egg. Just as NYC has more than one tunnel connecting the island of Manhattan to its outer boroughs and neighbors, most women have two fallopian tubes, so theoretically there is an alternate route for the sperm and egg to connect. The problem is, tubes are meant to serve the adjacent ovary, so if an egg is ovulated from the right ovary, it's very hard for the left one to pick it up if the right tube is blocked. While the opposite tube can, on occasion, grab an egg from its partner, the rate of pregnancies achieved from an ovary with a blocked tube does decline.

Treatment for tubal disease is largely dependent on if one or both tubes are out of commission. Years ago, tubal surgery was a possible fix, but the blockage could still recur. It is no longer commonly performed, as rates of ectopic pregnancy are high, candidates are limited based on age, sperm quality, presence of other pelvic pathologies, tubal length, and IVF success rates are so high. (When I was a fellow at one of the largest programs in the country, we did not do one such procedure in three years!) Rather than treating tubal disease with surgery, IVF is the best game in town, is typically covered by insurance for medical necessity, and success rates are high. In such cases, I think of myself as a matchmaker: I'm just connecting a good egg with some good sperm. Once they're all in the room together—inside the lab and then the uterus—the star-crossed lovers connect and sparks are likely to fly! In some cases, tubes need to be taken out before an embryo is put back in in order to increase the likelihood of implantation.

UTERINE PATHOLOGY: I am biased as an obstetrician/gynecologist, and also as a woman and mom, but to me, the uterus is by far the most awesome organ in the body. Its ability to grow and shrink throughout the menstrual cycle, pregnancy and the postpartum period is no less than astounding. Prior to puberty, it measures around 3 to 4 centimeters, and then it reaches about 36 centimeters when a woman carries a full-term pregnancy. Don't you agree that is astounding? Unfortunately, along with that elasticity and incredible capacity to nurture an embryo come some potential issues, as the uterus is a prime culprit in the "whodunit?" infertility game.

Some uterine problems that can make achieving pregnancy challenging include fibroids, polyps, adenomyosis, scar tissue or other adhesions, and congenital malformations. If surgery is required, which is frequently the case, it may be via a vaginal, laparoscopic, robotic, or abdominal approach.

It can be minimally invasive or more complex, but either way the uterus is like Rocky and can, in most cases, get back in the ring with a return to normal function after the requisite rest.

ENDOMETRIOSIS: Truth be told, "endo," as it is commonly called, is my second least-favorite diagnosis after unexplained infertility. Endo is a condition in which tissue similar to the uterine lining grows in places outside of the uterus, like on the ovaries, tubes, bladder, intestines, the abdominal cavity, pelvic ligaments, and even the lung.

It is a fairly common disease affecting about one in 10 women, and most women are diagnosed in their 20s or 30s during their prime childbearing years. Research suggests that 25 to 50 percent of infertile women have endometriosis and that 30 to 50 percent of women with endometriosis are infertile. Worldwide, 190 million reproductive-aged women are impacted by this condition. If the numbers seem astonishing, I am right there with you: The Big E (no relation to the Big C, cancer) is a biggie. The true prevalence of endometriosis is nearly impossible to quantify because diagnosis requires surgery and a pathologist's review of excised tissue. Most women will never get that far and therefore go undiagnosed. While the only way to officially diagnose endometriosis is to perform surgery, remove the abnormal tissue, and send it to a pathologist for review, a strong suspicion can be engendered by taking a really good history, doing a thorough pelvic exam, or seeing endometriomas (ovarian cysts) on ultrasound.

Much like cancer, endo is classified into stages based on the prevalence of aberrant tissue: minimal, mild, moderate, or severe (or stage I to IV). Unlike cancer, however, the stage of endometriosis does not always correlate with the symptoms. In addition to causing infertility, it frequently causes painful or heavy periods and pain with sex, urination, or defecation. Severity of symptoms does not correlate to stage of endometriosis; severe symptoms can arise from mild endo, and a patient with severe endo may exhibit mild symptoms. Some women report no symptoms at all and only discover incidentally when undergoing surgery for another cause that they have endo.

There is almost no reproductive condition that engenders more debate, disagreement, and confusion than endometriosis. Despite decades of research into what causes it, how it causes infertility, how best to treat it, and the long-term consequences of having it, endometriosis remains an enigma to many. The potential causes of endo are as varied as the impact it can have on a woman's life. Scientists have suggested it may be caused by retrograde menstruation, which is when blood goes backward from the uterus into the fallopian tubes and the pelvic cavity rather than forward and out the cervix. Or perhaps it's caused by lymphatic spread in a faulty immune system that fails to recognize the abnormal cells outside of the uterus; or coelomic metaplasia, in which cells that line the pelvis, ovaries, bowel, and bladder transform into endometrial cells. Genetics are also a factor, as those with an affected first-degree relative have between a seven- and tenfold increased risk for developing endometriosis. Some scientists have speculated that diet, environmental factors, or the use of exogenous hormones like estrogen can also contribute.

Endo causes infertility in a myriad of ways, including distorting normal pelvic anatomy or pelvic adhesions that make it even more challenging for the fallopian tubes to capture the egg, for the egg and sperm to meet, and for an embryo to get back into the uterus.

Endo can also increase the concentration of bad actors that cause inflammation. Would you want to take a swim in pea soup? Didn't think so. Same goes for an egg, sperm, and embryo, which is why the environment endo creates can make it hard (or nearly impossible) for pregnancy to occur. Endo has also been suggested to alter antibodies and white blood cell levels that can impact the endometrium's ability to accept and allow an embryo to implant; reduce ovarian reserve; impact egg quality; and affect hormonal function.

I could (but won't) write a whole book on endo and infertility, so this serves as a brief window into the subject. Treatments vary based on the patient's pain level, stage of endometriosis, and future fertility plans, but almost always involve medication, surgery, IUI, IVF, or a combination. While medical treatment works well to relieve the pelvic pain caused by endo, it does nothing to improve or treat infertility. That is when IUI or IVF comes to the rescue.

ENDOCRINE SYSTEM: Think of the endocrine systems as an orchestra composed of the brain, the pituitary gland, and the endocrine organs. The brain, more specifically the hypothalamus, is the conductor; the pituitary is the concertmaster; and the ovaries/testicles, thyroid, and adrenals are the strings, brass, and percussion. They all must perform their job well and at the appropriate time to create a beautiful sound, or in this case, to successfully release an egg, form an embryo, and achieve a pregnancy. Abnormality or pathology at any level can derail the whole symphony, shattering dreams of playing at Carnegie Hall.

To get a bit more specific, hormones are chemicals that are released into your blood and send messages between organs. The brain is the leader that kicks off most systems, including puberty, the menstrual cycle, and ovulation, by releasing gonadotropin-releasing hormone (GnRH). In terms of reproduction, this hormone travels to the pituitary and tells it to make other hormones, FSH and LH, which then travel to the ovaries, signaling them to make estrogen and progesterone, to grow and release an egg, and to develop the uterine lining. The pituitary, which plays telephone with the message sent from the brain to the ovaries, can be the source of problems when there are tumors, called adenomas, that can impact ovulation, causing irregular menstrual cycles and infertility. Depending on size, they can also cause headaches and visual changes. Prolactinomas, which are the most common benign pituitary adenoma, lead to increased secretion of the hormone prolactin, which prevents the hypothalamus from releasing GnRH. If the conductor, a.k.a. the hypothalamus, cannot lead the orchestra, the rest of the instruments stay quiet. That is what happens when lack of GnRH leads to no FSH or LH, and, in turn, the ovaries do not release estrogen or allow an egg to be developed and released.

The thyroid, which can be implicated in numerous health issues like weight fluctuations, sleep disturbances, GI issues, skin and hair changes, joint and muscle pain, memory problems, and changes in heart rate, also plays a prominent role in fertility. Thyroid disturbances, whether too much (hyperthyroidism) or too little (hypothyroidism) secretion of the hormone thyroxine, can impact ovulation as well as the ability to get and stay pregnant. With one in eight women having thyroid issues, they are 10 times more likely than men to be adversely impacted by this gland. Severity of the disease can vary, but even mild or subclinical cases can affect ovulation and require treatment. Aside from affecting the ability to get pregnant, thyroid disease, when untreated or poorly treated, has been associated with poor obstetrical outcomes such as pregnancy loss and pre-term delivery.

Like the thyroid, adrenal glands are another part of the endocrine system located far from the ovaries yet connected to fertility. Situated on top of the kidneys, the adrenals are integral to hormone production for some of the heavyweights: testosterone, cortisol, aldosterone, estrogen, and progesterone. They take their signal to play from the orchestra's bigwigs, the hypothalamus and the pituitary, and then get to work creating the building blocks that impact fertility, specifically ovulation. Diseases impacting adrenal function are less common than the thyroid, but no less disruptive to the various systems that lead to a pregnancy.

Treatment for most endocrine causes of infertility involves oral agents and/or hormonal injections, all aiming to retune the orchestra, bringing homeostasis and harmony back to the body's most incredible symphony.

CERVICAL ISSUES: When it comes to infertility, the cervix is lower down on the list of causes, but it can still be a culprit. Think of Club Uterus as the hottest spot in town, and the cervix is the bouncer who stands strong at the door, protecting any riffraff from coming in and stumbling out. If the bouncer does her job right, she allows the baby to pass from the uterus into the world at the opportune time. ("You are 10 centimeters dilated" may be what you hear when it's time to start pushing, referring to how much the cervix has opened.) If the cervix dilates prematurely, it can lead to preterm delivery.

The cervix also is charged with producing mucus that facilitates sperm transport. When the cervix is not producing mucus or has become narrowed, medically known as cervical stenosis, infertility can arise. By bypassing the cervix with an IUI, the sperm and egg can connect more expediently.

PELVIC ADHESIONS: Scar tissue is a natural part of the body's healing process that can occur after an injury, surgery, or infection. No different than scar tissue that can build up on any part of your body, bands of scar tissue that stick together in the pelvis can form an adhesion. The obstacle course that sperm and an egg go through to find each other and fertilize is already pretty intricate, so when you add an adhesion into the mix, it is like a roadblock or pothole that makes everyone's job a little harder or prevents organs from functioning normally, which can result in infertility and pain.

Pelvic adhesions can arise from a myriad of causes, including sexually transmitted infections like gonorrhea, chlamydia, and other pathogens that cause pelvic inflammatory disease (PID), pelvic or abdominal surgery, endometriosis, or inflammation. Even a previous C-section can cause scarring and adhesions that make getting pregnant thereafter more challenging.

In most cases, depending on the extent of the scar tissue, surgery is usually the go-to treatment.

MALE FACTOR INFERTILITY: Fertility is not just a female problem, despite centuries of that default assumption. Nearly one-third of infertility cases are caused by issues with sperm, and approximately 20 percent of all infertility diagnoses result from a combination of male and female factors. Abnormalities ranging from low or no sperm production, reduced or absent sperm motility, abnormally shaped sperm, blockages in the male reproductive organs, dilated veins in the testicles, hormonal imbalances, and genetic aberrations can impact male fertility. Along with abnormalities in sperm production and function, testosterone levels can be negatively impacted. Treatment can range from oral medications, IUI, IVF, or IVF/ ICSI to surgery or donor sperm, depending on the primary cause of the problem.

Patient POV

Tallulah, 50

Before I married my husband, I knew that he had very low or no sperm count. He and his first wife had tried to get pregnant unsuccessfully, so I was the beneficiary of the testing they had done prior. As soon as we got engaged, we saw an infertility specialist that a friend had recommended, and we approached sperm banks to get the ball rolling. I was 35, so we wanted to be aggressive and not waste time.

When choosing sperm, we wanted a donor who resembled my husband, so we considered features like height, hair color, eye color, and body type for the first pass. Once we narrowed the options down, our second pass was more about values and lifestyle, like someone who was educated and had similar interests. The donor we ended up choosing was in graduate school, thought family was important, was captain of one of his high school's sports teams, had a nice smile, and was described as affable. I will never know what is nature versus nurture in terms of how kids become who they are, but ours are pretty academic, athletic, and personable, so maybe we tipped the scales by picking the sperm we did. I should have bought enough sperm the first go-round to ensure that we could use the same donor for more than one child, but I didn't think of it. We got lucky that when we went back to the sperm bank after having our first child, the same donor was still available, so both our daughters have the same genetic father. Once in a while I worry that I didn't know enough about our donor's health history, especially mental health, but then I remember that no partner comes with a perfectly clean slate. It's not like finding out your spouse had a great-grandparent with depression would be a deal-breaker when falling in love and then starting a family.

IVF involves a lot of money, time, unknowns, and hope. It's extremely stressful to invest so much when there are no guarantees, but I never lost sight of how fortunate we were that science could help us become parents. We told our kids very early on about the process that led to building our family. Our girls feel like ours as much as if my husband's genes were in the mix.

CHROMOSOMAL ABERRATIONS AND GENETIC MUTATIONS: Select chromosomal rearrangements and genetic mutations can impact the production, viability, and quality of eggs or sperm, which can cause infertility. Individuals whose chromosomes, either partially or fully, have gone rogue and decided to swap places or partners in the chromosome lineup can cause big problems. In the case of chromosomal aberrations, the individual who harbors the swap-up or mutation may be none the wiser until they attempt to achieve a pregnancy. Their lineup may be off but they have not lost or gained an extra player; they are what we call in medicine, balanced. Unfortunately, their gametes have too many or too few players on the chromosome field and are referred to as unbalanced. This gain or loss of genetic material can translate into infertility and/or recurrent pregnancy loss. Examples of autosomal chromosomal aberrations include balanced translocations such as reciprocal translocations or Robertsonian translocations. In both conditions, the individual who harbors the mutation has not lost or gained any genetic material, hence the term balanced.

The good news is that the less-than-ideal rearrangement of chromosomes will have no impact on the affected individual's day-to-day life. The bad news, however, is that this rearrangement can go unnoticed until pregnancy is attempted and infertility or recurrent pregnancy loss occurs. At that point, chromosomal aberrations can be diagnosed with a blood test that reveals an abnormal karyotype (an individual's complete set of chromosomes) in one of the intended parents' egg or sperm source.

Specific genetic mutations affecting the X or Y chromosomes as well as other mutations or abnormalities in genes on nonsex chromosomes can also cause infertility. For example, the FMR1 gene, which is located on the X chromosomes, can result in fragile X premutation syndrome. This abnormality can be detrimental to the production of viable eggs and healthy pregnancies. Some people who carry the premutation suffer from serious infertility as well as a significantly higher incidence of early menopause. It is also not uncommon for some people who harbor the mutation to give birth to children with severe disabilities. Additionally a deletion on the Y chromosome, such as microdeletions in the AZFa, AZFb, or AZFc region, can lead to oligo or azoospermia. (If it sounds like I'm speaking an incomprehensible language, no need to get bogged down by the details. Just trying to give an overview of how various mutations in genes can lead to developmental problems or infertility.)

Lastly, individuals with medical conditions like CF that impact select genes can experience infertility. CF, specifically in men, can obstruct the release of sperm. Even men who do not have CF but carry one abnormal copy of the CF gene can experience infertility. In the majority of the cases pertaining to a genetic or chromosomal abnormality, treatment requires IVF to allow for preimplantation genetic testing.

CANCER AND CANCER TREATMENT: Cancer and the treatments used to eradicate these malignant cells, like surgery, chemotherapy, and radiation, can impair fertility. Whether it is the removal of critical reproductive organs, the development of scar tissue in the pelvic cavity, or the early exhaustion of gametes, treatment for cancer can take a toll on every aspect of one's life, including family building. I know firsthand how badly cancer sucks, but it sucks all the more so when it affects your reproductive organs or future fertility. Oftentimes, young cancer patients are faced with decisions like beginning treatment immediately versus delaying to first preserve their fertility. Recently, oncology practices began partnering with fertility clinics to ensure timely referrals for patients who want to explore fertility preservation options, egg, sperm, or embryo freezing, before cancer treatment is initiated. However, cost and access can still be a barrier to initiating care.

Patient POV

Jane, 48

I was 37, and my marriage was rocky. The kid thing kept coming up, and I was like, *How can we have a baby when I don't even know if the marriage will last?* We were on vacation, trying to figure things out, when I noticed some blood in my bathing suit top that had come out of my nipple. After a mammogram, ultrasound, biopsy, and MRI-guided biopsy, I was pulled into the scary room where I was told I had breast cancer. Ultimately I got a mastectomy, and there was a chance I needed chemotherapy, which would likely make me infertile, so I started thinking about egg freezing. I ended up not needing chemo but decided to move forward with egg freezing. I had worked in finance, so I had money saved and could afford to pay out of pocket.

I got only three eggs and was so upset. I felt like such a failure. I had lived a pretty healthy life but started to blame myself for cancer and for only getting three eggs. Had I partied too much? Been too stressed out? Waited too long? Self-hatred consumed me along with fear that I had ruined my chances of having a baby. A year later, I was diagnosed with melanoma, and then a lump in my breast was discovered to be cancerous again. This time I did need chemotherapy and radiation, so first I did another round of egg freezing. I got zero eggs. I begged my oncologist to give me the time to do one more round of freezing with a different doctor, and thankfully it was Dr. Knopman who discovered I had been suffering from endometriosis my whole life. She also was perceptive enough to see that my marriage was not stable, so freezing embryos, which would be joint property, was off the table. We moved forward with one more round of egg freezing, and I got three.

I am now in remission, divorced, and thought about becoming a single mom by choice but then decided against it. I have an insanely busy career, I'm an aunt, a godmother, and if I end up in a relationship with someone who has kids, I can become a mom that way. I have come to peace with my decision not to use my eggs, but I don't want anyone else to feel powerless about their fertility while they are letting the word "cancer" sink in. I started a nonprofit called The Chick Mission, which supports young women with cancer by helping them preserve their option to become a biological mom in the future. We have helped women freeze thousands of eggs. There was a time when all the lights were out inside my head and heart, but now I am at peace. Tackling this inequity and ensuring others don't suffer indignity has healed me.

LIFESTYLE: From nutrition and smoking to stress and excessive drinking, the impact of lifestyle on fertility is hotly debated. You already know that I find advice like "Just relax and you'll get pregnant when the time is right," or "Have you tried cutting out gluten and dairy from your diet?" to be condescending, shame inducing, and ill informed. Since the dawn of time, people have gotten pregnant in the most untenable circumstances and unhealthiest situations. Nonetheless, lifestyle does impact our bodies, albeit in ways that can be hard to quantify when it comes to fertility. Smoking is the only social habit that has been consistently demonstrated to reduce one's fertility and hasten the onset of menopause. It is also clear that heavy alcohol consumption, drug use, poor diet, insufficient sleep, excessive caffeine, and exposure to toxins are not good for our overall health. If you came into my office telling me you get high often, love to party all night, subsist on sugar and caffeine, and never exercise, I would most certainly suggest lifestyle changes. Scientific evidence correlating them with infertility and the above behaviors is lacking, however, so I may couple such lifestyle changes with treatment. (I will not, however, recommend that a man change his type of underwear! There is very little evidence that a man's underwear significantly changes his sperm count.)

The impact of weight, in both extremes, can cause irregular ovulation, a decline in natural fertility rates, lower sperm count and quality, and decreased success following infertility treatment. Unlike the American ethos, more of something is not always better. Especially when it comes to health, overdoing anything can be consequential. Too much exercise, too much food, too much food restriction—and the list goes on—can all culminate in not-too-good outcomes for your fertility. Modifications in lifestyle as well as medical and surgical management to treat those who are severely underweight or overweight can improve fertility outcomes.

RECURRENT PREGNANCY LOSS (RPL): While more of a symptom than a cause of infertility, RPL makes this list because it strongly suggests that there is an underlying fertility problem. All aspects of infertility can be disheartening, but in my clinical experience, going from the high of conceiving to the low of losing a pregnancy can leave patients with a painful sense of whiplash and heightened concern about long-term inability to conceive. Telling a patient the pregnancy has not progressed, that the fetus does not have a heartbeat, or that the pregnancy tissue is being passed is one of the hardest things I do. Most patients tell me they know the news just by looking in my eyes.

Clinically recognized pregnancy loss occurs in approximately 15 to 25 percent of pregnancies, but this number is probably actually higher because many women who test positive for pregnancy at home never even make it to see a doctor before losing the pregnancy. Such early losses that are not recognized by a clinician would not be included in the aforementioned clinical loss stat. Case in point: In the 1980s, a landmark Columbia University study analyzing daily urine specimens of 221 women who were trying to conceive found a total rate of pregnancy loss of 31 percent following implantation. Given that modern-day pregnancy tests are even more sensitive than they were in the '80s, if this study was repeated today, the number of pregnancy losses would likely be even higher.

While one miscarriage can be heartbreaking, it does not necessarily mean you are headed down the path of a formal diagnosis and treatment. Sporadic loss occurring before 10 weeks of pregnancy is typically the result of random numerical chromosome errors (like Trisomy 21 or Monosomy 10) and is often a result of advanced female age due to compromised egg quality. In such cases, treatments like IVF with PGT-A are usually successful in achieving a healthy pregnancy. Around 20 percent of all clinically recognized pregnancies end in miscarriage, but recurrent pregnancy loss as a result of causes other than sporadic chromosomal anomalies is a distinct disorder that affects fewer than 5 percent of women.

Sources differ on the exact number it takes to be diagnosed with RPL, but after two or three clinical miscarriages, a visit to the fertility doctor is warranted. A battery of tests can indicate if the suspected cause is structural chromosomal abnormalities within one of the intended parents, APS (antiphospholipid syndrome), uterine anatomical abnormalities (fibroids, structural malformations, polyps), hormonal or metabolic disorders (thyroid disease or diabetes), inherited thrombophilias (clotting disorders), autoimmune disorders, sperm fragmentation, infection, or lifestyle. Despite the lengthy list of options, more than 50 percent of recurrent pregnancy loss cases do not have a clearly identified cause. After rounds of testing, no solid answer about the underlying cause of miscarriage can be frustrating, but the good news is that nearly 60 to 70 percent of couples who experience RPL will go on to have healthy pregnancies.

UNEXPLAINED INFERTILITY: Ovulation is occurring, egg quantity is adequate, tubes are open, uterus is clear, semen analysis is normal . . . and yet a couple, in the midst of their childbearing years, cannot conceive after having unprotected sex at the right time for many months. What gives? Unexplained infertility, referred to as UI, affects about 20 percent of couples who seek treatment. When I tell a couple they may have UI, I often say, "If you're staring at all my degrees thinking, *Lady, you went to school for umpteen years, spent countless hours training, ran all these tests on me, and you still can't figure out what the problem is? I'm outta here*, I get it and can't blame you!" Not getting a specific diagnosis and treatment plan is a hard pill to swallow. We all want answers and action steps, especially when it comes to something as important as having children. When the expert has no specific expert advice to offer, it can be frustrating to say the least. The diagnosis of UI can only be made after an evaluation has been completed and all puzzle pieces are fitting.

Most of the causes of UI are not unknown diseases but diseases that our modern-day diagnostics cannot pinpoint. UI may arise from conditions such as reduced egg or sperm quality that cannot be identified, "silent" endometriosis (not visible on ultrasound), implantation failure, inability of a sperm to fertilize an egg (this cannot be seen on a routine semen analysis), autoimmune diseases, and genetic mutations. After ruling out all the other possible causes, treatment usually begins with oral medication and IUI. If three or four rounds of this treatment are not successful at achieving a viable pregnancy, a move to more aggressive options like IVF is recommended. Every patient is different, as some may opt for IVF from the get-go, depending on age and ideal family size, and some may never choose that route.

A Dietitian Weighs In

From gut health and inflammation to hormones and blood sugar levels, our bodies are complex, with numerous internal systems and external factors at play. Infertility is a medical disease, as I have made clear, one that often requires medical intervention. That said, a healthier body can lead to a healthier pregnancy because the systems in our body often work together.

According to Alli Magier, a dietitian who specializes in fertility, women should have nutrition and lifestyle choices top of mind even before trying to conceive.

"Poor diet, smoking, lack of exercise, and a thyroid that isn't regulated can have a negative effect on every system in your body, including fertility," says Magier, a mom of two. Rather than depriving yourself or becoming restrictive, Magier suggests asking what you can add to your diet to make it more nutritious and anti-inflammatory.

Antioxidant-rich foods that she typically recommends include vegetables, leafy greens, berries, citrus fruits, and colorful vegetables like carrots and bell peppers. "Half of the food on your plate at any given meal should be vegetables," says Magier, who prefers organic when possible in an effort to reduce exposure to possible endocrine-disrupting chemicals.

For clients who are hoping to conceive in the near term or already struggling to, she focuses on foods rich in vitamin E, such as wild salmon, almonds, kiwi, beets, nuts, seeds, and collard greens. Magier also recommends plant-based foods high in iron and folate, like beans and lentils, as well as healthy fats and protein, which can be found in avocado, wild salmon, sardines, walnuts, pasteurized eggs, grass-fed meat, and organic plant-based products like tofu.

"Nutrition-based interventions, even as simple as eating more plants, can get a body out of survival mode and help address underlying chronic issues that can impact fertility," says Magier.

Selecting a Doctor and Clinic

As I tell my daughters (or as *Wicked* told them in song), sometimes you have to just close your eyes and leap. Infertility is common, you are not alone, and there are numerous treatment options, so take the first step of choosing a clinic or a physician. What follows is quite similar to the process described in Chapter 4 for patients who are proactively preserving their fertility, although for infertility treatment there are some variations in what to consider.

In some areas, fertility clinics are nearly as prevalent as pharmacies in a strip mall, while other parts of the country are "fertility deserts," where access to care is out of reach for millions of people who seek it. Luckily, telehealth can be an option. Obviously you cannot get your ultrasound performed remotely, nor can an embryo be fertilized over a video call, but it is worth noting this option as a possible first step for you. Some fertility benefits providers like Progyny, Maven, or Carrot offer consultative services to members, as well as a list of recommended clinics along with reviews.

As much as it pains me to say this, keep in mind that fertility can be a big business, and it's one that grows bigger with each passing year. Some specialists will work with women in their mid- to late 40s to freeze eggs, even though the doctors know full well that these efforts will most likely be futile. Are these businesses taking advantage of these women or just doing everything within their power to try to help? Do the patients truly understand what the odds are but decide to move forward nonetheless? I do not know. But I do know that a desire to be a parent can be so overwhelming that whatever one is being sold can seem like a good idea to buy. Continued regulation and oversight of the industry is required to ensure that all practitioners are providing high-quality medicine, and it is also imperative that patients do their homework. Whom you decide to partner with on your fertility journey can be the difference between walking away with a baby versus walking away with nothing more than debilitating bills.

Patient POV

Anne, 39

After several years of marriage, I had my IUD taken out when I was 31. We were so hopeful and excited about having kids, but my period never came. After seeing my gynecologist and an endocrinologist, I found out I had an autoimmune thyroid issue called Hashimoto's. I started IVF at a highly regarded fertility clinic and, long story short, it was hell. In our first cycle we made embryos but decided not to have them tested. Because of my husband's Catholic upbringing, we were cautious about playing God too much, and since I was pretty young, we didn't think it was necessary. My first pregnancy was ectopic, and I ended up in surgery with my right tube removed. I had several more transfers, some of which failed, and one successful pregnancy that I miscarried at nine weeks. We had gone through all of my embryos and I was broken. You feel like your whole life is over because you can't do the most natural thing that you expected your body to be able to do.

    I knew I needed to make a change, so I switched to a new fertility practice and also started seeing a functional medicine doctor and a reproductive immunologist. I wanted to throw everything I could at the problems, whether I was addressing the root cause of my Hashimoto's, caring for my liver and gut health, or making my home and body a friendly environment for a future baby. Unlike my former doctor, Dr. Knopman didn't keep saying "Let's try again" to what clearly wasn't working in hopes that at some point it would just work out.

She listened, she assessed the whole picture of my health, and she was open-minded about new treatment strategies. I hope other women also advocate for themselves as CEOs of our own health. Accept nothing as normal and take stock of your body.

I had so much heartbreak along the way, but now I'm a mom to two healthy, happy kids who are 16 months apart. I'm not ready for another yet, but knowing that we have frozen embryos is liberating. So much about my fertility was out of my control, and now the ball is in my court. That's powerful.

Here are five considerations when selecting a physician and clinic for infertility treatment, many of which are similar to the guidelines I have offered previously for fertility preservation:

How long has the clinic been around, and what are its success rates?
Fertility clinics are popping up in some parts of the country more frequently than coffee shops or corner delis. Just because a clinic is new does not mean you should discount it, but my preference, when there is more than one option, is to go with a clinic that boasts high success rates over a good stretch of time. The formula for positive outcomes includes skilled practitioners, a high-quality embryology laboratory, and the use of novel technologies in a rapidly changing field. If a clinic is using outdated methods, that should be a red flag. Do a bit of research online with websites run by SART or CDC to see how a clinic's statistics compare nationally, and try a site like FertilityIQ to gather reviews or ranks of physicians and clinics.

Get practical. What are the hours of operation? How and when will you have access to a physician?
This may sound like small potatoes compared to whether a physician has decades of experience thawing and fertilizing eggs, but in actuality, a clinic's hours can have a big impact on the process. If you are a teacher who is in the classroom by 8:00 a.m., a clinic that does not take patients until after the school bell rings will not work for you. These morning slots are critical as they are when your blood is drawn multiple times a week. If the clinic is open early but a practitioner is not available until later in the day, that

may be a deal-breaker. Along those lines, ask who performs various duties so you are crystal clear about whether a trained specialist will be your point person or whether the person who answers the phone at the front desk is your primary contact. (The latter may be lovely, no disrespect! But, personally, I would want to ensure I had access to someone on the medical team, not an administrator, when it is time to review results, and that is the standard I hold myself to for my patients.) Will the physician be reachable directly by phone or via an app? How quickly can you expect to hear back? If time is of the essence and a two-week wait to speak or meet with a physician is standard, that may not be the right fit for you. What is protocol for emergency situations? Fertility treatment can be lengthy and disruptive, so do a little legwork to avoid the possibility of unnecessary roadblocks or logistical issues adding to the stress. Having all this information at the outset can also help you set expectations.

Who is on the team?

I am never so brazen to think that I have all the answers. I am only as good as my team, which includes capable (more aptly, badass) nurses, embryologists, surgeons, and other partners in medicine, such as oncologists, mental health providers, and minimally invasive gynecologic surgeons. On many occasions, there is a perplexing set of data that requires all hands on deck so that together as a team we can help build families using modern medicine. That is why I recommend that you find a physician who is well trained and confident yet eager to call on other resources when needed. When that happens, are those resources in-house? Do you see your MD regularly, and is that MD board certified? I hope so. Does the clinic have residents, fellows, physician extenders (physician assistants and nurse practitioners), and ultrasonographers? Who will be managing your care is an important piece of information to have from the outset. Some clinics are more staffed up than others, and the options in your area may be limited. Not everyone on your team has to be located under one roof, but having access to various players can prove critical. From the starting lineup to the backup bench warmers, find out who all the players are.

What practice style and bedside manner works for you?
You are not getting married to this clinic or practitioners, but you are potentially going down a long, intimate road together, so thinking of it like dating isn't too much of a stretch. Some physicians are reserved, while others are quite chatty. (You have not met me, but I am pretty sure you've figured out I fall into the latter category.) Some move fast, and others move slow. Some ring alarm bells after one failed round of IVF, while others patiently, methodically suggest next steps without a tinge of distress. Some communicate by phone, while others have online platforms. Some matter-of-factly tell you no eggs are viable, while others exhibit compassion and warmth. Some clinics resemble a factory, with patients shuttled in and out, while others offer a more personalized experience. A bond of trust is, of course, key. Do you feel comfortable when you walk into the office and a sense of assurance that your best interests will be served? Do you trust that the physician will level with you even if there is news you do not want to hear? A doctor who seems like they would sugarcoat difficult news could sour the relationship, so think about that in advance. You want a physician who is honest, straightforward, competent, compassionate, and any other traits that you value. You may not get everything you want in one clinic or practitioner, but ask questions so you can make an informed choice or, at the very least, be prepared for what lies ahead.

Consider cost.
At the outset of treatment, you have no way of knowing if you will be a one-and-done patient or if you are in for the long haul, so ask for a complete financial breakdown of possible treatments. Do they take insurance? Is there a billing or finance team to answer questions as they arise? Do they offer payment plans? Are medications a separate cost or is there a packaged deal? If you need multiple cycles, can you buy in bulk like Costco? I do not know your specific financial concerns, so formulate the questions that are relevant to your circumstances and make sure you get answers that work for your budget and your goals.

Patient POV

Taylor, 45

Nobody expects to have a fertility issue when you're young, in love, and trying to start a family. There's no reason to think about it . . . until, unfortunately, there is. I was rounding the corner on my 30th birthday when I went off the pill. Month after month passed with no luck, and my OB-GYN told me to keep trying for a year. That was the first moment that I recall realizing I would need to advocate for myself and make informed decisions that felt right for me. What could be the upside in waiting to do a fertility workup? I initiated blood work and other testing despite my doctor's suggestion that I be patient.

We had several obstacles in the way and opted for IVF, which became a multiyear journey that ultimately led to our family of three healthy kids. I was told that the quality of the lab that our fertility doctor worked with was the most important factor to consider when selecting our team. The embryologist may have been the most skilled in the universe, I'll never know, but what came along with that lab was a clinic that made me feel like I was being treated in a factory. I'm not the touchy-feely type and never would have thought bedside manner was a big deal, but when I was pumped up on hormones, devastated by miscarriage, petrified I may never become a mom, and fighting with my husband because we each coped differently, a little TLC would have gone a long way. The process can be nerve-racking, and you can feel very alone and helpless. When doctors don't respond in a timely manner, a few days can seem like an eternity. Fulfilling my dream of becoming a mom was a long road, but we got there. I don't see why more couples don't find out about their fertility and any possible bumps they may encounter as soon as they tie the knot or even before. Information is power.

What to Expect

After choosing a practitioner and clinic, a consultation will include a review of your and your partner's (if you have one) reproductive, gynecological, medical, surgical and family histories. It is likely that your doctor will waste no time gathering data by running blood tests, including ovarian reserve testing (FSH, AMH), hormone levels (thyroid-stimulating hormone, prolactin), blood counts (CBC), blood type, infectious disease, and genetic carrier testing. If certain conditions are suspected, additional hormonal blood work may be ordered.

A pelvic ultrasound will allow your doctor to see the stars of the reproductive show: the ovaries and uterus. (No, we don't care or even notice if you haven't had a bikini wax or shaved your legs in ages. There are more important issues to tackle!) This noninvasive exam can reveal ovarian cysts, reduced egg quantity, fibroids, polyps, or the growth of pelvic masses. It is frequently possible to visualize the fallopian tubes on a pelvic ultrasound or more frequently on a FemVue or HyCoSy, but the best way to assess their condition is with a dye test called a hysterosalpingogram (HSG). The safest and most reliable time to perform this specialized X-ray is in the first half of the menstrual cycle. An iodine-based contrast dye is injected into the cervix, with the aim of making its way through the uterus, fallopian tubes, and into the pelvic cavity. (Heads up: Some patients find taking ibuprofen beforehand to be helpful, as it can be somewhat painful.) By outlining the inside of these organs, the test shows if tubes are blocked and where a possible blockage, like a fibroid, polyp, scar tissue, or uterine malformation, may be. If the dye cannot get into the uterus and out of one or both tubes, then b-i-n-g-o, a cause of infertility is identified. Once the mystery is solved, treatment can begin.

No fertility workup for a heterosexual couple would be complete without a semen analysis. "Trust me, I know my guys can swim," is not an acceptable response from a male partner who is reluctant to have his ejaculate examined. A semen analysis is a laboratory test that evaluates parameters such as volume of the ejaculate, the quantity of sperm, the motility and progressive motility of the sperm, and the morphology (i.e., shape) of the sperm. A two- to five-day period of abstinence prior to the test is advised.

To recap, the basic diagnostic checklist for an infertility workup includes:

1. Consultation including a thorough medical history (including a partner if there is one)
2. Physical exam + pelvic ultrasound
3. Blood work (AMH, FSH + Estradiol, LH, TSH, prolactin, testosterone), CBC, genetic carrier screening
4. HSG
5. Semen analysis

If pathology is noted or strongly suspected, your fertility doctor may add on tests like a hysteroscopy, a laparoscopy, vaginal cultures, uterine biopsies, thrombophilia panel, markers for autoimmunity, or other diagnostics to identify underlying problems that can lead to infertility. If male-factor infertility is suspected, a referral to a urologist is in order along with a physical exam, hormone panel, Y chromosome genetic testing, testicular ultrasound, and in select cases sperm DNA fragmentation testing. The leave-no-stone-unturned attitude is often embraced while trying to get to the root of the problem, even though some tests could lead to a wild goose chase without a clear-cut path for treatment.

I strongly recommend that once all of the test results are back, you connect directly with your physician, either in person or virtually, to review results. A doctor who thinks an email with some numbers listed in a column suffices is not, in my estimation, the kind of partner you want for this journey. It is like a red flag early on when you're dating; if a physician doesn't take the time to go over the results in depth, particularly when there may be concerning data to review, I would move on. (Or maybe that's your jam! It's your call, but know what you are getting and make sure you are on board.) Bedside manner matters. This relationship can be long, and it's important to create a productive, comforting dynamic and communication style that works for you.

The Infertility Treatment "Ladder"

I think of infertility treatment as a ladder. You start at the bottom and gradually, methodically climb your way to the top, with each step offering a different treatment modality. The transition between each rung is not necessarily linear, and you may end up going up and down the ladder more than once in either direction. Depending on your age, diagnosis, number of kids desired, medical history, genetic makeup, and insurance coverage, in the words of House of Pain, you may be asked to "Jump Around" in order to reach the destination of parenthood. On this ladder, skipping a rung or two is no big deal nor even necessary unless your insurance company mandates otherwise, as some coverage requires a specific order for patients to ascend and descend the stairs. There is no maximum number of trips up and down the ladder, and each rung can be physically, emotionally, and financially depleting.

Each rung of the ladder represents a different modality aimed at reaching the desired goal of parenthood. Notice I said "parenthood" and not "pregnancy," because not every rung or course of action involves conception or pregnancy—for example, adoption. As outlined in the sections that follow, the lowest rung of the ladder is unprotected intercourse (if there are two people with opposite gametes), and if any step is unsuccessful or not applicable, there are others to step on. There is no specific or methodical order for ascending or descending, so think of it more like a choose-your-own-adventure story that you experience in tandem with physician guidance. I delve further into specific types of treatment in the subsequent chapter, but this is the overview of the ladder.

TIMED INTERCOURSE

Plain and simple, have consistent unprotected sex on the days that you are more likely to get pregnant. Sperm can live in the reproductive tract for five days, and the egg lives for an additional 12 to 24 hours after ovulation, so by "timed" I do not mean timing it to the minute. If you have sex on a Saturday and then ovulate on a Tuesday, the sperm is still there! For some couples, the process can suck all the fun and pleasure out of sex, but you do not have to be so formulaic in order to get results. While many of my patients use apps, ovulation sticks, or temperature charts, I believe they are often unnecessary, anxiety provoking, and in some cases even unhelpful. My recommendation is to get acquainted with the length of your menstrual cycle because if you are regular, you will ovulate around the same time every month. No matter how long the first half of any menstrual cycle is, the second half is 12 to 14 days. Ovulation occurs right between these two phases, known as the follicular phase and the luteal phase, so the formula is length of cycle minus 14 to determine ovulation. If your cycles are 30 days, then by subtracting 14, it's likely you ovulate on or around day 16 (30 minus 14). If your cycles are 26 days, subtract 14 and it is clear that around day 12 is go time. If your cycle is longer at 35 days, expect to ovulate on or about day 21. (Occasionally the luteal phase can be shortened, in which case the whole algorithm is slightly off, but most of the time the formula works.) Once you have figured out your ideal window for unprotected sex, go for it. If your schedules do not match up and you can only have intercourse on one day of the whole cycle, go with the day before ovulation. Being early is better than being late because the egg only survives for 12 to 24 hours post-ovulation, while sperm has a five-day lifespan. A mentor once taught me, "The guy should always be waiting for the girl," so let the sperm wait and give the egg priority.

INTRAUTERINE INSEMINATION (IUI)

Whether because the male partner has ejaculatory dysfunction, a couple is same-sex, or there are geographical limitations, placing sperm directly into the uterus at the time of ovulation is a viable option. This technique is primarily geared toward couples who have not been able to expose eggs to sperm on a routine basis, in which case additional treatment may not be required. While some couples may try a turkey baster at home to shoot ejaculate into the vagina, an IUI in a clinic entails separating the sperm from the rest of the ejaculate through a high-speed spinning process. Then, the fastest moving sperm are placed into a catheter and ejected into the uterus. Think of IUI as giving the sperm a head start by bypassing the vagina, or as an assist to ensure that the egg and sperm are in the same place at the same time, on or around the day of ovulation.

ORAL MEDICATIONS

If ovulatory dysfunction is the sole cause of infertility, oral medications such as clomiphene citrate (Clomid) or letrozole (Femara) are frequently used to induce ovulation. If a 28-year-old woman is not ovulating because she has PCOS, for example, a doctor might prescribe letrozole or clomid. Clomid was the go-to medication in this category of drug for nearly 50 years, and letrozole has taken the lead more recently because of reduced side effects coupled with improved success rates and lower chances of multiple gestation. Each has three dosing options, so a physician may try the same medication at a higher dose if needed, or switch to the other oral medication over time if needed.

ORAL MEDICATIONS + IUI

Clomid and letrozole actually work double duty. I think of them as showing up to a ball with a change of clothes at the ready so they can make the night a two-for-one. Clomid, a selective estrogen receptor modulator, and letrozole, an aromatase inhibitor, are used to induce ovulation in women who do not ovulate regularly. For women who ovulate but still experience infertility, clomid and letrozole are used to cause "superovulation," the release of more than one egg. They achieve these two goals by different mechanisms, but the end product is the same: ovulation of more than one egg. If you buy more than one lottery ticket, your chance of hitting the jackpot increases. If you release two eggs rather than one, you have double the chances of getting an egg fertilized. Data shows that the addition of IUI to the oral agents in couples where the female partner is ovulating but pregnancy is not occurring is key. Even if diagnostic testing shows semen to be normal, the oral medications alone do not appear to be enough to provide a real bump in success rates for such couples. The combo of an oral agent and an IUI has been shown to offer increased success over simply trying on their own in couples with conditions such as unexplained infertility, male factor infertility, endometriosis, and modest declines in ovarian reserve. Clomid and letrozole rarely lead to the release of more than three eggs or to multiple gestations, especially in couples where the female partner is ovulating. When they do, the physician should have a thorough conversation about risks and may recommend pulling the plug and canceling the cycle due to risk of conceiving a high-order multiple pregnancy (HOMP).

GONADOTROPINS + TIMED INTERCOURSE OR IUI (GND/IUI OR OVULATION INDUCTION/IUI)

These treatment modalities involving fertility-stimulating hormones, FSH and LH, combined with timed intercourse or IUI used to be a go-to. These days, like my hair's side part and my 1980's shoulder pads, they are far less prevalent. In women under 35, multiples were common, and in women over 35, miscarriage was not infrequent. Rather than taking daily hormonal shots and visiting the clinic every other day for the modest success rates these treatments offer, many women are opting for IVF. If IVF is not an option or insurance companies mandate this rung of the ladder before leaping to IVF, shots of FSH and LH are given for approximately eight days, then a trigger shot is given when the follicle size and estrogen level increase appropriately, followed by intercourse or an IUI in the next 36 hours.

IVF WITH FRESH EMBRYO TRANSFER

Many people do not realize that the treatment regimen for the first half of IVF, egg freezing, and embryo freezing involve the same protocols for the most part. The process of injecting fertility hormones daily, morning blood tests, vaginal ultrasounds, and timed egg retrieval is the same no matter what steps the patient intends to take thereafter. It is in the second half of the game that paths diverge depending on if the patient is implanting an embryo via IVF or opting to freeze either an egg or embryo. For IVF with a fresh embryo transfer, after the eggs are extracted, they will briefly hang out in the laboratory inside the media, which is the fluid that fosters growth of the embryo by providing the necessary nutrients until the timing is right to connect with sperm. Depending on sperm parameters and previous IVF history, fertilization is attempted either by insemination (thousands of sperm are placed atop of one egg and the fertilization happens on its own) or ICSI, which is a fancy way of saying sperm is injected into the inside of the egg using a microscopic needle. While I am a firm believer in the benefit of embryo biopsy, genetic testing, and embryo freezing, not all clinics across the country offer such testing. Some clinics prefer to analyze embryos on day three or day five, and then transfer them into the uterus fresh, rather than frozen, based on their morphological appearance. Unfortunately, an embryo may look high quality but could harbor incorrect genetic profiles or have other issues, so with fresh IVF transfer, miscarriage due to chromosomal abnormalities is a higher risk.

IVF + EMBRYO BIOPSY + FROZEN EMBRYO TRANSFER

As we work up the ladder, IVF with all the frills (e.g., embryo biopsy and embryo freezing) is more invasive and expensive, so it is not typically the standard first-line treatment for most couples. It is, however, the most successful treatment for the majority of infertility diagnoses using autologous gametes (one's own eggs and sperm), particularly when a frozen embryo that has undergone biopsy is transferred.

When freezing and testing an embryo before transfer, think of it as a game where the referee calls a timeout, giving the team time to evaluate strategy and select the best players for the next play. In fertility treatment, having a window for an extended embryo culture and genetic testing gives your team the best chance of sinking a three-pointer for the W. The highest pregnancy rates in fertility medicine are achieved with a single tested embryo transferred in a frozen embryo cycle. Not only is it beneficial for the embryo to undergo genetic testing, but by pressing pause, there is also time for the body, specifically its hormonal milieu and ovary size, to return to baseline before the embryo is placed inside the uterus. Pregnancy and neonatal outcomes have been shown to be better in frozen rather than fresh embryo transfers. That is because hormone levels can stabilize and, as demonstrated in large studies, creating an intrauterine environment is a better place to grow and nurture the embryo and resultant fetus.

Female age is a huge factor, but most people require several rounds of IVF before achieving success. On average nationally, it takes around six IVF cycles to have a successful live birth. Based on my clinic's average, I tell patients to buckle up and lock in for three cycles, though of course that number depends on how many children someone intends to have, their health history, age, and more. That's a reasonable start, as it can be a huge psychological hurdle to think about more than three. Not everyone can afford six, therefore I believe that after three is a good time to reassess the impact on your body and what other strategies may be worthwhile to consider. We learn a lot from previous IVF cycles, such as the best mixture of medications for each body, the best day to extract eggs, how one reacts to specific hormones, and more.

One large study of approximately 150,000 women who did about 260,000 cycles found that one cycle has a 29.5 percent success rate, cycles two through four have a 20 percent success rate, and then by cycle six it jumps to about 65 percent. The more cycles a woman undergoes, the greater the chance that a live birth will occur because it is basically a numbers game. I think of it like my daughter's attempt to score a goal in soccer: The more she shoots, the more likely she is to score.

DONOR GAMETES

For women whose eggs are not viable, for men whose sperm is problematic, and for same-sex couples of either gender, using a donor gamete—either an egg or sperm—is an ideal option. Jumping to this rung on the ladder can be challenging for people who expected parenthood to be genetic. In my experience, even those of us with the least bravado harbor visions of passing on our genetics to our children. A whole chapter devoted to the ins and outs of this avenue to parenthood is coming up, but for now, know that it is one of the rungs on the ladder when other applicable methods have failed.

GESTATIONAL CARRIER, A.K.A. SURROGACY

For some people, getting pregnant is not problematic, but carrying the pregnancy is. This might be the case for women who have uterine malformation, uterine fibroids, uterine scar tissue, cervical insufficiency, or a contraindication to pregnancy. Following IVF to obtain embryos from the intended parent(s), the selected embryo(s) is transferred into the uterus of a surrogate, who carries and hopefully gives birth to a baby for another person or couple. In my opinion, giving another woman an egg or the use of her uterus is one of the greatest gifts one can offer. This rung on the ladder is not stepped on as often as some of the others because of the limited number of available surrogates, legal restrictions, and cost, and its medical necessity is not as prevalent as that of other conditions.

SURGERY

For patients with fibroids, uterine scar tissue, congenital uterine anomalies, or ovarian cysts, the removal of such pathologies may be necessary before pregnancy can be achieved. In such cases, surgery—abdominal, laparoscopic, robotic, or vaginal—is the treatment of choice to restore functionality to the specific organ in the female reproductive system that was impacted. Route and type of surgery will be selected depending on the pathology, its location, and the patient's medical and surgical history. There are select cases in which surgery can treat male factor infertility as well, like varicocele repairs or testicular sperm extraction. While surgery, either on the female or male, can have a positive impact on restoring fertility, frequently IUI or IVF are required to further improve success rates.

ADOPTION

I have minimal expertise with this rung of the ladder because it is not a medical treatment like the other steps (with the exception of timed intercourse, which some people end up treating like a medical procedure). For some people the journey toward parenthood begins with adoption, as I recently had a patient who adopted her first child and came back a few years later to freeze embryos and achieved a pregnancy. Conversely, I have a patient whose first child was biological, and for their second child they fulfilled their dream of adopting a girl from China. In many cases, adoption is a choice people make when other avenues of family building were unsuccessful.

As the science behind treatment for infertility advances, some steps of the ladder will get a revamp. Multi-embryo transfers, daily intramuscular shots, exploratory abdominal surgery, and postcoital cervical tests (microscopic evaluation of the cervical mucus following intercourse to check if the mucus is healthy) are rungs of the ladder that are no longer recommended, but some clinics may still offer these procedures. Also, tubal surgery to fix damaged fallopian tubes, particularly distal tubal blockages, is no longer a preferred treatment option. (Most doctors trained after the early 2000s were never taught how to even do these.) While my BFF, who is a fashion stylist, tells me to hang on to my skinny jeans because everything old comes back in style, these procedures have become mostly obsolete. I mention them here only so that if they are recommended by your doctor, you should do your homework to better understand why.

Alternative Treatments

While acupuncture and Chinese medicine have been around for ages, in the last several years there has been an influx of alternative treatment options for infertility. From herbal and nutritional supplements like CoQ10 to dietary modifications, off-label medications, and infusions and injections like PRP (platelet rich plasma), the number of products claiming to improve fertility—without much reliable or reproducible data as backup—is enough to keep your social media feed populated for days.

I value teamwork, and I'm keenly aware that I'm never a one-woman show, nor should any physician be. I give it up to my Eastern medicine colleagues who have been practicing medicine, including acupuncture and herbal medicine, for centuries longer than Western practitioners like me. If a patient is struggling to get pregnant, alternative modalities of treatment should not be in lieu of what a reproductive endocrinologist or other medical fertility specialist offers, but part of a holistic approach.

How About Acupuncture?

As touched on in Part 1, some patients couple medical treatment with an acupuncture regimen. Although there are no definitive recommendations supporting the use of acupuncture to improve patient outcomes, I am a fan of an integrative approach. Mary Sabo, whose Chinese medicine and acupuncture practice is dedicated specifically to reproductive care and fertility support, suggests having a meeting (or "intake session") with an acupuncturist prior to any treatment. If preparing to freeze eggs, she recommends getting started two to three months prior to the retrieval cycle, and during a cycle she typically meets with clients twice weekly.

Just as a regular fitness regimen can lead to positive changes in the body, acupuncture can stimulate the parasympathetic nervous system, help prioritize blood flow to the reproductive organs, and reduce inflammation, Sabo explains. Acupuncture needles are extremely thin, about the width of a strand of hair, and most often painless. For some patients, the primary benefit of acupuncture is support managing stress and anxiety, and others report positive impact on sleep, energy, menstrual cramp intensity, PMS moodiness, and cycle regulation. Herbs and supplements, as well as diet and lifestyle modifications, may be recommended to optimize your overall health and body chemistry. Not all Western medicine practitioners are in the know about Eastern medicine and holistic approaches, but I still recommend open communication so that all your specialists are on the same page and working together to help you get pregnant.

I am skeptical of some additions to the fertility marketplace. There is a growing business of fertility "coaches," "experts," and "platforms," some of whom may be well trained while others may have no credentials and offer unsubstantiated clinical advice, tools for "ovarian rejuvenation," or promises of healthy embryos. I hope there will be more research-backed data as the market evolves, rather than just a strong foothold in chat groups that can spread quickly. In general, I recommend knowing the credentials of any "experts" offering guidance, and I think the cost of any offerings should be clearly laid out. (Same goes for medical treatment, obviously.) I understand the desire to cover all bases, especially if a long journey of infertility has left you wanting to throw all kinds of paint at the wall. I do not believe nonmedical additions to your regimen are typically harmful, but I suggest that you go in with eyes wide open, protecting both your expectations and your pocketbook. Modifying your diet and taking supplements may give you a sense of control in an uncontrollable process, but understand that even if you can control what you eat, you cannot control if an embryo will implant. Staying hydrated and taking a prenatal vitamin are worthwhile additions to your regimen, but they have no ability to fix uterine scar tissue if that is your underlying issue. Infertility is a disease, and all the kale in the world cannot change what you were born with, what time has done, or your partner's ailments. Nonetheless, a healthy body makes for a healthy pregnancy, so I am all for maintaining a healthy lifestyle, all the more so when trying to conceive or carrying a pregnancy.

In my in-person consults, now would be the time that I say something along the lines of, "I just talked a lot and realize your head may be spinning. What questions do you have for me?" I would also acknowledge with eye contact and empathy that I know experiencing difficulty getting pregnant downright sucks. Unfortunately, I cannot ask you the same, but instead I can assure you that this ladder of infertility treatment is a darn sturdy one. If you ever feel stuck on a rung you wish you weren't on, can't fathom mustering the strength to take a step up or down, or feel like the whole ladder is about to tip over, know that there are so many options that have been proven to be successful under all kinds of circumstances. Remember the classic board game for kids, Chutes and Ladders? If you feel like you are slip-sliding down a massive chute, like the dreaded spot 87 that lands you flat on your butt back at space 24, I am here to remind you that there is no one way to get pregnant. If being a parent is what you want and you are open to making that happen, perhaps in a different way than you may have anticipated, you will get there one way or another.

The Biggest Little Things You Can Buy or Borrow: Donor Eggs, Donor Sperm, and Surrogacy

As you know, the modern-day family is no longer composed of a mom, dad, 2.2 children conceived through intercourse, and a dog—nor should it be. Admittedly, I did not intuitively understand this or come to this realization overnight. When I delved into the ins and outs of gamete donation as a medical student on my Reproductive Endocrinology and Infertility (REI) rotation, the concept of borrowing or donating precious reproductive cells to build a family befuddled me. I sat next to my mentor as he counseled a couple struggling with infertility to consider egg donation, thinking: *Who was going to donate an egg to them and why? Would the patient and donor ever meet each other? Would they want to? What were the finances involved, if any? Would they tell their child one day? Was this couple devastated, hopeful, or somewhere in between?* Using a third party for an egg, sperm, or as a surrogate defied the fairytale image I naively had of what becoming a parent would look like, notions that had been ingrained in me probably since I played with dolls as a little girl.

As I've explained throughout this book, millions of individuals have become parents using donated eggs, sperm, embryos, or gestational carriers. When one or more of the pieces of the infertility puzzle is missing or impaired, whether by choice or not, how kick-ass is it that third-party reproduction exists—that humans are willing to provide each other with tissue to create life! If a woman falls in love at 38 and moves quickly to have kids with her male partner but discovers her eggs are no longer viable, she can go to an egg bank and create one or more embryos to build a family. It never stops astounding me even though it is part of what I do day in and day out. A single woman may decide to stop looking for Mr. Right and start picking out her ideal sperm donor on the path to single parenthood instead. What freedom! I am constantly in awe of the giving nature of others. (Surrogates and donors do get paid, but in my experience they are driven by altruism as well.) Adoption is another possibility, particularly if a couple's IVF efforts are futile. This chapter explores these oft-used paths to parenthood, including the scientific, legal, logistical, financial, social, and psychological aspects involved.

Oocyte Donation: A Brief Timeline

The first successful human oocyte (developing egg) donation cycle was performed in Australia in 1983, followed by the first US baby born from donor eggs in 1984. Up until this innovation, individuals or couples who lacked viable eggs had only adoption as a path to parenthood. This scientific breakthrough entailed the donor having her ovaries stimulated to produce multiple eggs in a single cycle, extracting the eggs at the ideal time, fertilizing them with sperm (either a partner's or a donor's), growing the embryo in a laboratory, and implanting the embryo into the recipient parent-to-be's uterus. The recipient mother can gestate, give birth, and even breastfeed. If there is a male partner, then his sperm creates a genetic link with the child, but there is no genetic link between the recipient mother and child.

The technology for egg donation and IVF has improved dramatically over the last 40 years. Its usage has increased, particularly among mothers-to-be whose path to parenthood begins once their eggs are no longer viable and same-sex male couples, who could previously only turn to adoption. The most recent data from SART shows that there were approximately 20,000 IVF transfers using donor eggs in 2022, up from the previous year. There is no data about donor egg cycles globally, as not all countries have regulatory agencies that require reporting, but according to the International Committee for Monitoring Assisted Reproductive Technologies (ICMART), there were 161,139 egg donation transfers in 2018. Between 2018 and 2022, the most recent years for which SART reported data, there have been nearly 100,000 transfers using donor eggs. By some estimates, there are 1 million donor-conceived people in the United States, whether via sperm donor or egg donor.

Scientific advancements made the process of egg donation more successful over the years. Even if the donor egg comes from a healthy young woman, extended culture and embryo biopsy have become all the rage for donor egg embryos, yielding improved success rates across the board. The advent of donor egg banks played a massive role in making the procedure more accessible. Rather than the months it could take to find a fresh donor, stimulate her and go through the process, with a frozen cycle, the eggs are already frozen and at the ready. In the 2010s, companies like Fairfax EggBank, MyEggBank, and Donor Egg Bank USA allowed clinics, couples, and individuals to more easily access and identify donor eggs. Whereas previously options were severely limited, increased access meant that an aspiring parent-to-be could scroll through a database of thousands. A parent-to-be could pick his or her desired egg donor on a Friday and have the eggs shipped to a fertility clinic by the following week for fertilization within days.

As with other aspects of ART, celebrities have played a role in normalizing gamete donation. Some celebrities who have used donor gametes or surrogacy, according to various news outlets, include Mariah Carey, Neil Patrick Harris, *NSYNC's Lance Bass, Camille Guaty, Cheryl Tiegs, *Shark Tank's* Barbara Corcoran, Sarah Jessica Parker, Marcia Cross, Jesse Tyler Ferguson, Ricky Martin, and Sir Elton John. Sometimes people, including celebrities, are more forthcoming about using a surrogate than they are about whose eggs were used. The former is, of course, visible to the world, while the latter can be a more private decision.

Patient POV
Emilio, 52

After I met my husband, we started to get all the mysteries ironed out of how to have kids if you're not in a male/female relationship. It seemed so overwhelming and expensive. The doctor helped by putting it into steps instead of thinking about the process from beginning to end.

When we were sent to get our semen frozen and tested, my husband was worried there would be something wrong with his sperm. It turned out I was the one who had a problem. As a cyclist for many years, my sperm were affected by testicular trauma. I was able to get some shots to improve semen count, and both of us were ultimately able to freeze our sperm. As the freezing process was concluding, we found a donor who met our criteria. She donated 26 eggs; I fertilized half, and my husband fertilized the other half. After all the eggs were tested, we found we had four viable embryos with my sperm and eight with his. We froze all of them.

Then we were put on a waiting list for a surrogate. We were on vacation when we got the call that a surrogate was ready for us, but we were not financially ready at that moment. We decided to hold off. By the end of the summer, we went back on the waiting list, and six months later we met our surrogate over FaceTime. She was great. We watched the transfer with the catheter going into her uterus with Embryo A and Embryo B, one of each of ours. Both took.

We had fraternal twins, a boy and a girl, who are now six years old. I don't know if every parent feels this way, but six years later, we still can't believe we are parents. We got everything we wanted and then some! It's not a far-fetched dream if you just take it step-by-step.

Using a Donor Egg

Frequently, those who turn to egg donation have tried IVF unsuccessfully or are same-sex male couples. Egg donation is a logical next step for couples who are emotionally, physically, or financially depleted from failed IVF cycles, as they often are hoping to use their remaining resources for a treatment option that would offer a higher chance of success. Oocyte donation is also used to prevent passing on heritable conditions in cases where couples do not want to do IVF with PGT-M (pregenetic testing for monogenic conditions) or for whom it is not possible. Egg donation offers success rates that approach 50 percent nationwide, and in select clinics that number is even higher.

Making the leap from autologous oocytes (your own eggs) to donor oocytes (eggs from a third-party donor) can be challenging. The ASRM recommends and it is also my personal practice to have all my patients considering oocyte donation undergo an evaluation and counseling by a skilled mental health professional before embarking on the process. When I sit with a couple that is contemplating it, I pull out pen and paper and draw a tree diagram. I like the image of a tree because the trunk and deep roots symbolize the foundation of a family and the depths of the bond, while the branches, representing a growing family, help prospective parents understand the different options that lie ahead of them.

Just like a matchmaker trying to produce a love connection, donor egg agencies, companies, and clinics offer eggs from individuals of all back-grounds with all kinds of traits that may be desired by the recipient parents. Donor egg banks source eggs from across the country, but not every box on your wish list may get checked off. Typical considerations can include height, eye color, hair color, and ethnicity, and I've had patients focused on academic credentials or athletic abilities. I even had one patient who wanted a ballroom dancer—and she got an egg from one! Some women try to find a donor who resembles them physically or has similar personality traits, but keep in mind that the perfect donor does not exist. Consider making a list of nonnegotiables versus nice-to-haves as a guide throughout the process.

While many people have donated blood, very few of us have or will donate a gamete. I have the utmost respect for those who do. It is a decision that comes with a lot of thought, some risk, counseling, and legal represen-tation. While such women are financially compensated, the money is not, in my opinion, commensurate with their efforts to give tissue that provides the building blocks for a family.

The first decision when selecting an egg donor is whether it will be anonymous/nonidentified/nondirected or known/identified/directed. This may sound like semantics or word soup, but it is actually a critical distinc-tion. Historically, egg donors, like sperm donors prior, were classified as anonymous, so the identity of the donor was not revealed to the recipient parents or future children. Such anonymity could be maintained with a high degree of certainty in years gone by. Now, however, with direct-to-consumer genetic testing, ubiquitous social media, facial recognition technology, and technological advances that allow us to connect with people across the globe instantaneously, the classification of anonymous or nonidentified is difficult, if not impossible, to ensure. Thanks to companies like 23andMe, AncestryDNA, or MyHeritage, among others, it is estimated that millions of Americans have their genetic information stored in privately owned and unregulated databases. As the at-home DNA testing technology continues to proliferate, identifying gamete donors and children born from donation will likely become even easier. As such, the term *anonymous* is, at best, misleading, and it has been replaced by the label of "nonidentified" or "nondirected." When eggs are nonidentified, the individual providing the eggs is not known to the recipients. Such eggs are typically sourced through a donor egg agency, an in-house clinic egg donor program, or a donor egg bank. Even when the process is deemed nonidentified or nondirected, certain banks will provide parents some degree of identification should they desire at a later date to initiate contact. The policies and practices of specific banks must be clearly communicated to both parents and donors before the donation.

When the donor is identified to the recipient parents, that is called a known, identified, or directed process. The donor may be a relative like a sister or cousin, a friend, or an acquaintance, with or without a genetic link to the future parents. Such donations are significantly less common than nonidentified, understandably so, given the magnitude of the relationship and the complexity of the process. In my own practice, no more than 10 percent of egg donations are directed.

Ideally, egg donors are healthy women in their prime reproductive years of 20s or early 30s without a personal or family history of serious medical conditions. All donors should be fully counseled on the risks and benefits of ovarian stimulation and egg retrieval, including legal counseling. The donors and their eggs go through a screening process, including medical, reproductive, and family history, so that hereditary diseases or genetic abnormalities can be identified and prevented from being passed on. Ovarian reserve testing, genetic carrier screening, infectious disease testing, and psychological counseling are all essential components of the selection process. Infectious disease testing, as mandated by the FDA and Department of Health and Human Services (HHS), must be performed at select times to ensure the accuracy of the results. The screening also includes a physical exam and a questionnaire about travel, sexual activity, transfusions, tattoos, piercings, and exposures to toxins. Select high-risk activities, such as ear piercing and tattoos lacking sterile conditions, do not prohibit donation but cannot be performed within a year of donation to prevent the transmission of infectious diseases. A positive gonorrhea, chlamydia, or syphilis test requires documented treatment and a year interval between positive test and donation. Individuals that test positive for HIV, Hep B, Hep C, and West Nile Virus are excluded from ever donating eggs. The screening process in the majority of facilities is thorough, so if you are on the receiving end of an egg, you can rest assured that no corners were cut to secure good eggs.

The going rate for an egg donor in the United States is approximately $10,000 to $12,000 for one cycle, but there is a range. I know a Harvard Medical School student who was recently offered $150,000 for her eggs; she declined before finding out if that fee was for one or more cycles. I also know of a couple who paid $250,000 for their egg donor, a beautiful, Ivy League–educated medical resident.

Fresh versus frozen is another decision for egg donor recipients to consider, though that was not always the case. Prior to the development and refinement of oocyte vitrification, all egg donation cycles were fresh. In this process, an egg donor's ovaries are stimulated for approximately nine to 12 days in a preparation process that mirrors what a woman going through IVF would undergo, including hormonal injections, ultrasounds, and blood work. After the eggs are retrieved and then fertilized with sperm in a fresh cycle, the resultant embryo is either transferred or frozen. The egg is never frozen on its own, so the first time any cells hit ice is after the embryo is created. If genetic testing is desired, the embryo must be frozen and transferred into the intended mother's uterus thereafter.

In most fresh egg donations, the eggs are allotted to one individual or couple, or they are split between two individuals or couples. With a fresh donation, recipient parents-to-be will frequently have a surplus of eggs and/ or embryos, as donors routinely produce 20-plus eggs, and in most cases the recipient or recipients have access to all of them. By freezing multiple embryos, the recipient has the option down the road of trying for multiple children that are genetic siblings.

Fresh cycles still exist, but they are no longer the default. Once the egg freezing and thawing process advanced with the technology of vitrification, combined with the advent and proliferation of frozen egg banks, donor egg cycles using frozen eggs became more common. In 2022, the number of frozen donor egg cycles outnumbered fresh egg donor cycles nearly three to one. Egg banks revolutionized donation by offering decreased wait times for eggs (because the eggs are already primed and ready for purchase) and decreased cost (nearly half of what a fresh donor cycle costs). Rather than all of a donor's eggs going to one or two couples, they can be divided into packets or lots of between five and seven eggs for use by multiple desiring individuals or couples at any point in the future. Although the success rates from frozen donor eggs still trump many other fertility treatments, success rates with fresh eggs are higher. Here's why: With frozen eggs, if the recipient buys only one lot, she has access to fewer eggs, around five to seven, than the likely 20-plus eggs that could be retrieved in a fresh cycle.

While many other countries maintain national donor registries and mandate that egg donors be legally identifiable to both recipient parents and offspring once the child reaches adulthood, the United States does not have a national registry, nor are there regulations that stipulate what or when the parents of donor-conceived children should disclose. The ASRM Ethics Committee encourages parents to disclose such information to their children at a point in the future they deem appropriate, and many mental health providers share the belief that nondisclosure violates a child's autonomy. Given the rise in direct-to-consumer genetic tests, unplanned disclosure can occur frequently. Ultimately, any decisions rest with the parents.

Patient POV

Leanne, 54

I was in my late 30s when I got married, so I was a little bit worried about my fertility. We got checked out and found out my husband's sperm had reduced motility. We were going to do artificial insemination, but right before starting, my FSH was too high. Only then did the doctor tell me that the chances of getting pregnant with my own eggs was about 5 percent, so he recommended IVF with a donor egg.

As a woman, you think you're supposed to be able to have babies and breastfeed and go through the whole process. I felt so let down by my body. It really affected my self-esteem and self-worth. It also put a damper on our sex life. Before trying to start a family, sex was for pleasure, but then it became all about getting pregnant. Once that couldn't happen, I didn't see the purpose of sex anymore.

Our doctor had in-house egg donors that were a lot less expensive than going to an outside company with exorbitant fees. We found a donor with a good health history who looked like she could be my little sister. My husband and I are both fairly intelligent and wanted our kids to have a good shot at success, so we asked about the donor's GPA, which wasn't included in her bio. We decided to move forward with the first cycle and got a decent number of embryos, but with every day that passed, some of them would not make it. We put in two embryos, but I didn't get pregnant. Weeks of a deep depression followed. Our next round using frozen embryos didn't work. By then I was almost 40, and I refused to plan a celebration because I was in a dark place.

I needed to keep moving forward or the sadness would be unbearable. We ended up choosing a very cute 21-year-old with a good health history. This time, we got healthy embryos and one took! As soon as our little boy, Jack, turned one, we transferred another embryo and ultimately completed our family with our daughter, Ella. We chose to donate the rest of our embryos to science.

The Process: IVF Using Donor Eggs

After the desired eggs are selected, the sperm source fertilizes the egg in a lab in order to create an embryo, a process that mirrors IVF, albeit with a donated egg. If embryos are not being frozen or genetically tested, then putting them into the uterus requires synchronizing the recipient's uterus and the donor's egg retrieval cycle so the uterus is primed and ready to accept the developing embryos. In recent years, cycle syncing has taken on a new meaning as women modify exercise, diet, sleep, sex, or other life-style factors to best suit different phases of the menstrual cycle. Originally, however, it was what fertility clinics did to sync the recipient's uterus and the donor egg's retrieval cycle to the same stage to prepare for the transfer, so I now refer to it as OG cycle syncing. Given the rise of frozen embryo transfers, both in IVF and egg donation cycles, old-school cycle syncing has become less common, while cycle syncing to improve fitness outcomes is on the rise.

Before embryos can be implanted, the recipient's uterus needs to be cleared of any uterine pathologies such as fibroids, polyps, or scar tissue. Infectious disease screening of both the recipient and partner is required, and then, if the all-clear is given, it's go time. The uterus doesn't age like the ovaries, so if it receives a healthy embryo, it frequently delivers a healthy baby.

Co- or Reciprocal IVF

Prior to 2009, a same-sex female couple had to pick which partner's eggs to use to create embryos with a sperm donor. If they had more than one child, perhaps they would have the opportunity to use eggs from each partner, but for each child, a choice had to be made. In 2009, co-IVF or reciprocal IVF, a treatment that allows both members of a same-sex female couple to participate in the creation and carrying of embryos, was introduced. With this arrangement, one partner provides the eggs, and the other partner carries the embryo and births the baby, thereby allowing both parents-to-be to experience a biological or genetic bond to the child and contribute to the process.

Over the course of my career, co-IVF or reciprocal IVF has become quite popular with same-sex female couples. This is a relatively new addition to the family-building playbook, and there are no rules. In some partnerships, carrying a pregnancy is completely off the table for one woman. In other partnerships, providing an egg is not in the cards. Regardless of who does what, I always recommend that both partners undergo a complete fertility evaluation at the outset because game-time decisions or switch-ups are not out of the question. If a couple plans on having more than one child and having each partner play both roles, then age and ovarian reserve are primary considerations for who will give an egg first. Who is more likely to carry first (or at all) is often dependent on medical history and uterine pathology. For example, if someone has a large fibroid that must be removed and will require a six-month time-out before pregnancy can be achieved, it is likely that this person will provide her eggs first and carry second so her uterus can heal. While the egg and uterus lineup can change, in most cases with same-sex female couples having more than one child, the same sperm source is used so that all of the children share genetics. Sperm can be provided by an anonymous donation or a directed donor.

All Things Sperm

Exactly 100 years before the first baby was born from egg donation, in 1884, the first baby was born from a donor sperm insemination. The story of how this first birth via sperm donor came to be is unethical, even horrifying, but worth mentioning if not for shock value then certainly to illustrate how far the field has come. In Philadelphia, there was a couple having trouble conceiving. As was the default for millennia, the doctor assumed female infertility was the cause until he discovered that the husband was azoospermic, meaning his semen lacked sperm. This physician had the wife come in for, supposedly, a routine exam, and then, unbeknownst to her, placed her under anesthesia (using chloroform!) and inseminated her (using a rubber syringe) with sperm from a medical student (ostensibly the best-looking one in the hospital). Nine months later, she gave birth to a healthy baby boy.

After that late-19th-century occurrence, , it took another 65 years for scientists to lay the groundwork for the cryopreservation of sperm. The first baby born from sperm that was frozen and then thawed was in 1953. In

1964, the first sperm banks opened in the United States and Tokyo. Commercial sperm banks came into existence in the early 1970s, starting in New York and then followed by a surge across the country. Until the 1960s, donor-conceived children were considered "illegitimate," and the practice of donor insemination was deemed "adultery" on the part of the woman. In 1973, the Uniform Parentage Act was passed, stating that if a woman was artificially inseminated with donor sperm under a doctor's supervision and with her husband's consent, the law would recognize the nongenetic father as the natural father of the child. Also, the donor was relieved of any legal or financial obligations.

Given that the United States does not maintain a national donor registry, it is hard to provide accurate numbers of births using a sperm donor. For years, the figure used in published medical literature was that 30,000 to 60,000 births from donor sperm were estimated annually, but many have speculated that this underrepresents the actual number because so many donor-conceived births are shrouded in secrecy. Some estimates indicate that between 2015 and 2017, around 440,000 individuals or couples used donor sperm. In the United Kingdom, babies born from donor sperm have reportedly tripled from under 900 in 2006 to over 2,800 in 2019.

Picking a sperm source is a highly individualized decision, one that can hamstring even the most decisive, opinionated women. When patients ask for my input, I explain that I am partial to genetics and family history. A 6-foot-4-inch, blue-eyed college athlete would be a bonus, but for me, family history and genetics trump all. For some, particularly if the goal is to raise a Knicks center, height and athletic ability may very well be a prime consideration. I have friends who thought an Ivy League education and good looks were essential, and one patient who would only consider a concert pianist. As I said, this is an individual decision, and there is no right or wrong. It is simply my opinion, as a mom and as a clinician, that genetic history is of the utmost importance. While all sperm donors are screened for health and some banks have a more stringent selection process than others, I would recommend a donor with little to no family history of heart disease, cancer, dementia, mental illness, or other heritable conditions. Donors fill out extensive questionnaires to give color about their personality and values, and some include audio of their voices as well. I have had patients split hairs analyzing what a donor may have meant in an answer to a particular question about his priorities or preferences. I believe that our children's values are a product of how they are raised (nurture over nature), and for me, DNA is about tipping the scales toward a healthy child rather than trying to replicate any particular skills or traits.

Like egg donation, sperm can be identified or nonidentified, but in the United States it is far more likely to be nonidentified. Some banks may refer to these classifications as open versus anonymous, but the ASRM thinks anonymity is no longer accurate given the prevalence of genetic testing services and the ability to connect with possible genetic links globally (and nearly instantaneously). Open or identified is when donor-conceived adults can request contact with their sperm donor, whereas nonidentified or anonymous means there is no identifiable information at the time of the transaction.

In the early days, the majority of donor sperm inseminations were fresh, as practitioners and patients feared that frozen sperm would offer reduced success rates. Despite evidence that disproved this theory and the improved accessibility and breadth of choice that frozen donor sperm could offer, it was not until 1985 when the AIDS epidemic hit that protocols began to change. The American Association of Tissue Banks, FDA, CDC, and ASRM all recommended that only frozen semen quarantined for six months be used for donor insemination. Fresh donor sperm inseminations can still be performed on the down-low at home (I've heard stories of people using a turkey baster!), but they are not regulated or condoned by fertility clinics because they lack the requisite medical screening and legal counsel, and increase the overall risk of the procedure. The majority of sperm donations in the United States and globally are obtained by purchasing anonymous donor sperm from a sperm bank, and then it is primed for either insemination or an IVF cycle.

In insemination, which is frequently referred to as IUI, the sperm is thawed and then washed to remove substances like dead sperm cells, white blood cells, and prostaglandins, all of which can cause some intense uterine cramping. Like rinsing dirty dishes before they go in the dishwasher, sperm washing removes debris that does not improve the success of an IUI. Or think of a load of laundry and how you'd wash whites separately from colors. Sperm washing separates highly motile sperm from less motile sperm to improve the chance that the best sperm in the mix get a head start and are likely to finish the race. Around the time of ovulation, the sperm is washed and placed in a catheter that is inserted into the vagina, through the cervix, and into the uterus.

If IUI is unsuccessful or if IVF is advised as the first course of action, then you can think of the egg and sperm's first date as chaperoned by an embryologist in the lab with some options for how they meet up. Conventional insemination involves dropping thousands of sperm on top of an egg in hopes that one ambitious swimmer will penetrate the egg's outer surface. Many couples opt for ICSI instead, so their embryos can be genetically tested with the highest degree of accuracy. With ICSI, the first date is a bit more monitored, as an embryologist injects one sperm into the egg to increase the chance of successful fertilization. Theoretically, donor sperm, which is from young, fertile men, should be competent enough to achieve fertilization, but success rates still depend on the egg and other pieces of the fertility puzzle. Once fertilization is achieved, pregnancies with donor sperm, whether through IUI or IVF, are no more complicated than those achieved with autologous sperm.

Single Mothers by Choice

In my own practice, and especially since the COVID-19 pandemic, I have seen a significant rise in the use of donor sperm by single women, frequently referred to as "single mothers by choice" (SMBC). Not only did more women become single mothers, but they became so at younger ages than prior to the pandemic as well. As time dragged on throughout months of quarantine, many of my patients faced intense loneliness and isolation coupled with a heightened awareness of their impending infertility. In some cases, the pandemic got them thinking about their mortality and legacy. That is when, they tell me, the goal of motherhood crystallized for them, and the work-from-home lifestyle gave them the flexibility to follow through with single motherhood. This is a dynamic that played out far beyond my practice, as the biggest sperm bank in the United States, California Cryobank, noted a 34 percent increase in single women's requests for donor sperm between 2020 and 2021. According to Single Mothers by Choice, a national network of groups that provide support and advocacy for single moms, there was a "big rise in activity" as soon as the acute stage of the pandemic began to subside, at which point people who had reevaluated their circumstances and goals sought their resources. Today, Cryo, an international sperm bank, reports that 50 percent of their clients are single women, a significant increase from just a few years ago.

How the sperm fertilizes the egg, whether via IUI or IVF, depends on several factors mostly related to the woman, such as age, fertility history, gynecologic history, number of desired children, number of usable sperm vials, and insurance coverage. In my experience, it is common to start with IUI and turn to IVF only if IUI is not successful. Most women who opt to become an SMBC do not have a diagnosis of infertility and are using sperm that is high quality, so with two pieces of the puzzle in solid shape, success rates are high.

Patient POV

Alison, 48

The night of my 38th birthday, I had a freak-out. Thirty-eight was the arbitrary age I had chosen to pull the trigger and become a single mom if I wasn't in a relationship that was leading to kids. It was a last resort and the time had come. I mourned the loss of the life I had always imagined I would lead and decided to make the best of the situation by getting pregnant on my own.

I took a few single moms to lunch to better understand their experiences, and they provided me with some resources like sperm banks. I also went to see my OB-GYN to get a better sense of my fertility and what the plan for getting pregnant would look like. I used a sperm bank where you are able to see adult photos of the donors, which is rare, because it was important to me that

I found the donor attractive. I also considered intelligence and healthy genetics. The process was actually fun. Picking out a sperm donor was like online dating, except you didn't have to actually find a connection with the person. I went through it at the same time as another friend so we could collaborate and commiserate.

I had an amazing support system in place made up of close friends and siblings. I am pretty sure some of them thought I was being rash and crazy to do it, but they still supported me every step of the way. My insemination process had its frustrations but was relatively smooth. I had two chemical pregnancies and then the third insemination was successful. My pregnancy went well, and I was able to carry on with life as I had known it. Labor was brutal and breastfeeding is the devil.

I had always wanted more than one child, but I wasn't sure if that would be doable as a single mom. Unexpectedly, I got pregnant with an on-again, off-again boyfriend a bit over a year after having my daughter, and our son was born. I now live with and share both kids with my boyfriend. Anything can happen. My advice to other women is that if you are thinking of doing it and are financially stable and up for a lifestyle change, do it! You regret the things you don't do more than the things you do.

I am fond of so many of my patients for numerous reasons, but the women in my practice who become single moms by choice are exceptionally badass. They may have taken a winding road before they reached my office with clarity and purpose, but by the time we move the process along, it is palpable that they know what they want and are ready to go for it. Even when my patients think they only want one child on their own, we discuss buying enough sperm for a second child and freezing extra embryos in case they decide to give their child a sibling.

In an effort to teach my own daughters how much is within their control—so long as they take action—I often tell them, "Don't stop moving. Just keep putting one foot in front of the other." I tie my advice to my marathon running and their passion for volleyball and soccer, suggesting they can always stop for water breaks, which could mean refueling with support, compassion, and love, or maybe to shed tears. Then it's back to one foot in front of the other. Women who proceed to become an SMBC when that may not have been what they originally wanted are doing just that. (So are plenty of other people who dust themselves off and embrace a path they didn't expect, but I still have the utmost respect for SMBCs). They set their eyes on their goal and move toward it, often setting their lives up in such a way so that they have a network of friends or family to support them rather than a partner. Some of them may have wished for a partner, but rather than lamenting what is missing or letting society tell them to follow a formula that is not right or feasible for them, they hit up the sperm bank and make their dreams come true.

Traditional vs. Gestational Surrogacy

Surrogacy, when a woman carries and gives birth to a baby on behalf of another woman, is a practice as old as time that has recently become almost as prevalent in society as my kids calling me "bruh." Dating back to the Bible and Hindu scripture, women opted to "share" another woman, sometimes a servant, with their husband for purposes of childbearing, as seen in the cases of Sarah and Hagar, Rachel and Bilhah, and Balram and Rohini. Fast-forward thousands of years later, to when surrogacy was formalized in the first legal contract in 1976. As the first IVF baby was not born until 1978, this surrogacy resulted from an IUI, and she was not compensated for her service. A few years later, the first surrogacy contract stipulating payment for the surrogate was penned, and in 1985 a surrogate carried a pregnancy that was genetically related to both intended parents for the first time. This was a game-changer. By removing the genetic linkage between the surrogate and the baby, the field shifted from what we now refer to as traditional surrogacy to gestational surrogacy.

With traditional surrogacy, which is rarely practiced today, the surrogate is inseminated with the sperm of the intended parent. The surrogate not only provides her egg, and is therefore the genetic parent, but also gestates and delivers the pregnancy, so she is also the biological mother. Legally, however, that baby is not hers, as she surrenders parental rights to the intended parents at birth, and the intended parents gain custody of their child with a post-birth adoption to which the surrogate consents.

You may recall the famous case of Baby M, a seminal ruling in family law from 1985. Elizabeth and William Stern contracted with a surrogate, Mary Beth Whitehead, to carry and birth their child so that Elizabeth, who had multiple sclerosis, would not pass on her health issues. After fertilizing Whitehead's embryo with William's sperm and inseminating her via IUI, Whitehead carried the baby, gave birth to her, and then refused to honor the contract that required her to yield parental rights to the Sterns. Whitehead fled to another state, the Sterns sued, and they ultimately prevailed but only after a lower court's ruling was overturned. It wasn't until Baby M turned 18 that any of Whitehead's rights were terminated, and to this day, that case reverberates, including heated debates about whether surrogacy contracts exploit women for their uteri.

The Baby M case expedited the demise of traditional surrogacy, which most clinics, surrogacy agencies, and states do not allow. Rather, gestational surrogacy, colloquially referred to as GC (gestational carrier), is practiced routinely today, though it requires IVF, which is more involved and costly than IUI. With GC, there is no genetic linkage between the surrogate and the embryo. The gametes of the intended parents or donor gametes—but not the surrogate's—are used to create the embryo, which is then transferred into the surrogate. A contractual agreement must still be signed, and every state has different laws, but this relationship and the legalities are less complicated than traditional surgery.

While the intended parents can usually establish their parental rights before the baby is born, there is still the potential for disputes to arise. In 1990, a gestational surrogate refused to give up the baby after delivery. When the case went to court, the fact that the baby had no genetic connection to the surrogate helped the intended parents win, a reminder of a significant advantage of gestational surrogacy. Though each state's laws vary, gestational surrogacy contracts are now legally binding once the surrogate is pregnant.

Gestational surrogacy for a fee is not legal in all states. As of January 2025, paid gestational surrogacy is not legal in Louisiana and Nebraska. Legislation about surrogacy is still evolving, as New York did not allow paid gestational surrogacy until February 2021, at which point the Child Parent Security Act went into effect, which also made it easier for intended parents to obtain legal parentage. As recent as 2024, Michigan passed the Assisted Reproduction and Surrogacy Parentage Act, which ended the criminal ban previously placed on surrogacy. Clearly, each state has its own view on and treatment of gestational surrogacy, and beyond laws that entail black-and-white legalities, there are further intricacies that may make the process easier or harder depending on location. (I will not address specifics because the goalposts are constantly moving and changes to legislation are ongoing.) If you are planning to use a surrogate, make sure to know the laws in your state *and* the state the surrogate will give birth in. I also strongly recommend hiring a surrogacy lawyer to help guide you or connecting with a nonprofit that offers similar resources. Lastly, choose a clinic that is competent and makes you feel comfortable so that if you do hit any hiccups along the way, whether legal or otherwise, you are supported and in good hands.

Patient POV

Ashley, 50

In my mid-20s, I was on a third date with a guy I really liked when I told him I could be infertile because of childhood cancer. If that increased risk was a deal-breaker for him, I might as well find out before getting more serious.

"So we'll adopt," he answered, unfazed.

We ended up engaged, married, and in the office of a well-regarded fertility expert. Testing revealed that my eggs were fine, but my uterus was not. Radiation had essentially burned through and thinned sections of it, making it too dangerous for me to carry a baby. Having viable eggs felt like such a tremendous blessing that not being able to carry and deliver seemed like no big deal. I think it's all about expectations.

Finding a gestational surrogate became my full-time job. We came up with three requirements: someone who had been a surrogate before, had children of her own, and had a support system like a spouse or partner. We found a surrogate across the country and started the IVF process. I produced seven eggs, which created three embryos, two of which were strong enough for the transfer. We flew the surrogate out, and I was sitting right beside her when both embryos were shot into her womb. One of them took.

Shortly before the birth, there were a lot of logistics to take care of, like ensuring my name would be listed as the mother on all legal documents; finding a pediatrician in the birth state prior to discharge; and getting my own hospital room on the labor and delivery floor so I could stay over like any other new mom. Until I saw my daughter and held her in my arms, it didn't feel real. I could finally breathe after we flew back home with her and walked through our front door as a family.

We made a conscious decision to be forthright about her birth story. We couldn't have been more grateful and proud, and wanted her to feel the same way. Using her favorite activity as an analogy, I said it was like baking a cake: "Daddy and I were the ingredients, you baked in someone else's oven, and you were ready on your birthday!"

Surrogacy in no way defines her or us, but it has been a beautiful blessing.

Who uses a surrogate and why? Just as egg donors or sperm donors are called in when the intended parent's egg or sperm source has either been depleted, compromised, or never existed in the first place, gestational carriers come into play when the intended parent's uterus has issues or suffers from a medical condition that impacts their ability to carry a pregnancy. Whether congenital or acquired, medical conditions affecting the baby can make pregnancy impossible or pose a significant risk to the woman and/or the fetus. Also, some couples or individuals, such as same-sex male couples, single men, or transgender individuals (depending on if they have a uterus or desire to carry if they do), are biologically unable to carry a pregnancy. Also, in cases where multiple embryo transfers of high-quality, genetically normal embryos have failed without any clear reason behind the inability to implant and develop, a gestational carrier may be used.

As someone who has carried two pregnancies, albeit neither past 36 weeks, I can say with certainty that pregnancy can take an emotional and physical toll. I recognize that I say this from a privileged vantage as someone who could get pregnant and deliver my daughters, but since I live by the principle of honesty, I admit that I was not a fan of the process, which I went through while going through rigorous medical training and sleep deprivation. I would do it a million times over to have my girls, but my personal experience is part of the reason why I have profound awe for women who choose to be surrogates to help other women become mothers. In the words of Aretha Franklin: R-E-S-P-E-C-T.

Surrogates should be between the ages of 21 and 45 and have a stable family environment with a solid support system. They should have had at least one uncomplicated full-term pregnancy of their own, so carrying your baby is not their first rodeo. Conversely, they should not have delivered more than five children vaginally or three children via C-section. Like egg and sperm donors, the screening process for surrogates includes medical and obstetrical history, social assessment, infectious disease testing, and a psychological evaluation by a qualified mental health professional. Ensuring that all parties—the GC, intended parents, and fetus—have their interests protected and are set up for the arrangement to thrive takes an all-hands-on-deck approach by numerous experts, and then many clinics add on their own layer of approvals before accepting a surrogate. Keep in mind that when a clinic asks you to jump through hoops, it is to protect all parties' interests. If a GC is rejected by your physician, ask questions so you are fully kept abreast about the valid medical reasons that give your doctor pause.

The GC is not the only one to roll up her sleeves and come clean about her past, as the intended parents also undergo blood work, physical examinations, psychological counseling, legal meetings, and risk assessments. Such screenings must be performed on all parties prior to the extraction of the eggs, deposit of sperm, and creation of embryos, and they are done on a specific timetable that is dictated by the FDA and each state's health department. Given the complexities of these relationships, mental health providers and legal counsel who specialize in third-party reproduction are critical. I partner with my patients throughout all parts of the process and lean hard on these resources for aspects that are out of my league. It takes a village before the child is even born!

Prior to the embryo transfer, infectious disease blood work must be repeated on all parties. The FDA recommends a six-month quarantine between embryo creation and embryo transfer into a GC, at which point testing should be conducted again to ensure none of the parties carry a risk that was not previously evident. When it comes time to move forward with the transfer of the embryo, it is strongly recommended that only a single embryo be transferred.

I recently transferred an embryo into a GC for a patient who had frozen embryos with her husband after she was diagnosed with breast cancer. That cycle in 2018 was successful, leading to two healthy embryos. For seven years the couple saved money for a gestational carrier, a lovely woman from Houston who had a five-year-old son. After the transfer, my patient said she wanted to share something with the surrogate. A few weeks earlier, she had attended a Jewish funeral and participated in the tradition in which mourners place three shovelfuls of dirt into the grave, over the coffin. This is considered an act of kindness, a deed that can never be repaid, as the deceased is buried by those who loved them. My patient told her surrogate, "It occurred to me that I, too, will never be able to repay you. Thank you for carrying my child." We all started to cry tears of gratitude for human kindness. The surrogate is pregnant, and when the baby is born, whether a boy or girl, the name will be Emmett, meaning "truth."

Patient POV

Maya, 49

My fiancé and I were busy planning our wedding when I realized that I had missed a period. I took an at-home pregnancy test, and we found out I was pregnant. We were shocked but couldn't have been more excited. When we went in for our 12-week appointment, there was no heartbeat. All I had known about miscarriage was what I once saw in a movie. It never crossed my mind that it would happen to me.

By then we knew with all our heart that we wanted to have a baby, so after our wedding, we started trying again. I got pregnant very easily but miscarried at around 10 weeks. My doctor told me there wasn't a lot of research about why people miscarry; my eggs had just gotten older, he speculated, and I should not be concerned. After my third time getting pregnant and miscarrying, I saw a specialist who diagnosed me with Antiphospholipid Syndrome, which basically meant my immune system was attacking the fetus. My specialist put me on medication that enabled me to get pregnant and stay pregnant. My pregnancy was hard and I was on bed rest, but at 39 I had a healthy baby boy.

I tried following the same protocol when we wanted a second child, but I couldn't hold the pregnancy. No heartbeat. My entire life revolved around pregnancy-miscarriage-pregnancy-miscarriage, and at the same time I was building up a big business. Every trip to the bathroom was to see if I was bleeding. My body was so stressed and exhausted all the time. I was intent on proving to myself that I could do what I had been told my whole life every woman can and should be able to do: get pregnant and deliver a baby. I was in my 40s, and I knew I was running out of time.

Stop being greedy, I told myself, *you already have your miracle baby.* But I really believed I was meant to have a second child. We decided to do one last round of IVF with a new doctor and committed to surrogacy if we got any healthy embryos because it was no longer safe for me to get pregnant again. We got three good embryos and found a surrogate in Kansas; she is proof that there are angels in this world, people who just want to give the gift of family to others. It was the most magical experience of my life while my baby was incubating with someone else.

Our kids are now nine and four, and I am still close with the surrogate who completed our family. I now know it's a myth that women are told that you should be able to carry a baby. There's nothing wrong with you if you can't, and I wish I had given myself a little grace. You can be a mother in any way.

Embryo Donation

When an individual or couple undergoes IVF for any reason, it is common for cycles to result in the creation of surplus embryos because we never know how many embryos will be needed to create a family. Such embryos are often used to create genetic siblings, but even after a family is complete, some additional embryos may remain. Embryo donation refers to the practice of donating such embryos to other couples or individuals to help them build a family. Embryo donation is often perceived to be synonymous with embryo adoption, but the use of the word adoption in that context is incorrect. It's like Alanis Morisette's hit '90s song, "Ironic," with numerous lyrics that are not examples of irony. Rain on your wedding day can be annoying and unexpected, but it's not ironic! I love the song, but "a traffic jam when you're already late" is also not ironic. Likewise, adoption describes the placement of a child with a family after birth, so donating embryos to another couple or individual does not constitute adoption. According to the ASRM Ethics Committee opinion, "Adoption is designed to protect the best interests of children, and the term has a very specific legal meaning that applies to existing children, not embryos which hold the potential for life but are not rights-bearing persons."

Deciding what to do with unused embryos is a weighty matter. Many individuals pay annual fees for decades, ranging from $500 to $1,200, to keep their embryos in storage, which can be a way to avoid making a difficult decision. For those who do not want to discard their embryos or donate them to scientific research, there is the option of donating embryos to another individual or couple in need. While embryo donation is the least commonly selected option, it is now being performed more frequently than in years prior. In 2014, 1,058 donor embryo transfers were performed, and by 2022 this number had risen to 2,431. Most embryo donations are nonidentified or anonymous, and all include appropriate screening, legal consultation, and psychological counseling. An individual or couple in need of an embryo would select one at an embryo donation center, and then the donated embryo or embryos would be transferred into the uterus of the recipient. Historically, success rates have been lower than those of egg donation, with around a 40 percent chance of success per transfer cycle, in part because some couples who turn to embryo donation may have underlying fertility issues and because the highest-quality embryos are not necessarily the ones that are donated. Nonetheless, as IVF success rates improve, so do success rates tied to embryo donation.

Adoption

When counseling couples considering third-party reproduction, I always discuss adoption, even though it is not technically in my purview since it is not a medical treatment. Many couples or individuals consider adoption for family building, whether as their preferred method or after IVF is not successful. Any conversation about moving to a different rung on the ladder can be challenging, especially the rungs that involve offspring with different genetics, but adoption is a beautiful way to build a family while also offering a loving, stable home to a child who may not have one. I encourage those interested in expanding their families through adoption to seek out individuals, organizations, and support groups that are extensively trained in how the process works and knowledgeable about the laws or other protocols in your state.

Global Disparities

At 16 years old you can vote in Argentina, and it is legal to drink alcohol in Switzerland. Cross the border into France and you've got to wait until you're 18 to pick up a drink. In Belgium, tobacco is for sale to 16-year-olds, and in Japan, it is not legal until 20. In Canada, at 14 you can be eligible for a learner's permit, while 14-year-olds in the United States can only get behind the wheel legally in Arkansas and Alaska. Countries and states are vastly different in their laws, including governance and cultural norms pertaining to reproduction.

While egg freezing exists throughout the world, select countries have varying restrictions. In Saudi Arabia and China, egg freezing is only permitted for women with medical conditions, such as a cancer diagnosis. Some countries have age restrictions. The Netherlands require women to be under 40, France subsidizes egg freezing for women between 29 and 37, and Israel restricts access to women between 30 and 41 years.

Cross-border differences are apparent when it comes to gamete donations too. In the United States, donor-conceived children are not routinely permitted by law to have access to their donor's contact information unless the donor consents. Genetic testing kits that reveal ancestry may have made so-called anonymous or nonidentified donation difficult to keep that way, but legislation is aimed at trying. Many countries in Europe take the opposite stance. Sweden was the first European country to prohibit anonymous egg donation in 1984, and most other European countries that permit egg donation now require donors to consent to their identity being disclosed to any resulting biological children, thereby eliminating nonidentified donation. Spain, Greece, and the Czech Republic are in the minority with a law that guarantees donor anonymity beyond general information about a donor, and revealing donor identity is a serious offense. In Hungary, the egg donor must be a member of the infertile couple's family, while Germany, Switzerland, Tunisia, and Turkey prohibit egg donation altogether. Countries also differ in whether compensation is allowed.

The number of donations an egg donor can make also varies worldwide. In the United States, according to the ASRM, an egg donor can donate up to six times over the course of her life. Once six cycles are completed, she is not eligible to donate eggs again. In Canada and Mexico, the same norms apply, whereas in the United Kingdom, a donor's eggs may be used to create a maximum of 10 families, not including her own. In Spain, the magic number is six, with laws prohibiting a donor from completing more than six cycles or achieving six births. In Israel the limit is three egg donation cycles, with at least 180 days between cycles. In India, a donor is limited to just one cycle. In many countries, including the United States, a centralized registry of egg donors and donations does not exist, so it is nearly impossible to enforce recommendations or regulations within its own borders, and very little can be done to regulate international donations.

As for sperm donors, in the United States the ASRM recommends that sperm donors be limited to 25 births per population of 800,000. California Cryobank and Fairfax Cryobank, two of the largest sperm banks in the United States, set a limit of 25 to 30 family units. However, there is no national sperm registry, and families are required to self-report births, which can impact the reliability of data. The majority of European countries maintain a registry of all sperm donors and donor-conceived individuals, which helps ensure that donors adhere to limits. In the United Kingdom, a sperm donor can provide children for up to 10 families, in France this number is six, and in Denmark, a donor can contribute sperm for a maximum of 12 families. Sperm donors are compensated in the United States, but in most countries, including Australia, the United Kingdom, Spain, Mexico, and Canada, compensation is limited to reimbursement for expenses such as travel and accommodations. In select countries, such as Germany, egg donation is not legal but sperm donation is.

When it comes to gamete donation and surrogacy, there is extreme variability worldwide in terms of who can offer services, if they can be paid, and numerous other considerations throughout the process that may be monitored by various agencies or governments. Even within the United States, each state has different legislation, nuances, interpretations, and requirements and the rules both in the United States and abroad are changing regularly. There are only a few countries around the world, including the United States, Ukraine, and Russia, where compensation to donors is permitted. In most countries, including Greece, South Africa, Spain, Israel, and Australia, compensation is generally limited to expenses for inconveniences related to the donation process (e.g., travel, missed work).

Other than the United States, paid surrogacy is only permitted in a few countries, such as Georgia, Ukraine, and Russia. However, only the United States, parts of Mexico, and Colombia allow commercial surrogacy regardless of sexual orientation. Switzerland, France, Germany, and Italy prohibit surrogacy completely. In October 2024, Italy made it illegal for individuals to engage in international surrogacy, with a punishment of up to $1 million and jail time up to two years.

Regardless of the differing laws across the globe and within the United States that govern a rapidly evolving and politically charged field, it is clear that there are numerous ways to build a family. Some paths to parenthood may include potentially circuitous and hilly roads involving donor gametes or surrogacy, vital and miraculous feats of modern medicine that all adults and adolescents should know about. I have armed you with the basics of what using a donor egg, donor sperm, or a surrogate entail, but this is not intended to be a medical textbook, nor can I advise you every step of the way (unless you are my patient) if one of these paths is or becomes yours. Knowing when to move on from your own or your partner's eggs, sperm, or uteri to a donor or surrogate is not always clear. There are no flashing lights like at a railroad crossing indicating when it's time to pump the brakes on IVF or go full speed with egg donation. It is up to you and your physician to determine the best course of treatment, the appropriate timeline, and if there is a need to pivot to a different course at any point along the way.

CHAPTER 7

Fertility Misconceptions and Facts

IF I HAD A DOLLAR for every patient who walked into my office and eagerly asked for "the fertility test"—sure as the sky is blue that I could prick their finger or draw blood and then report back with clarity about just how fertile they are—I could spend at least the next decade offering reproductive care for free. There are as many myths surrounding fertility as there are motile sperm in an average man's ejaculate! (By now you know that means a lot.) There is almost nothing I have not seen, heard, been asked, or been told about fertility. Dr. Google, a relative of the old-school game of telephone, has allowed many myths and first-person anecdotes to practically become doctrine. If you want to understand modern-day fertility, it's time to replace misinformation that spreads like wildfire with fertility facts, the most up-to-date, easily digestible material that we all need to know. Infertility is a disease or condition with massive implications for millions of people, so it's high time to empower people to make smart choices and get the help they may need. In this chapter, I will address the most common misconceptions, pun intended, about fertility, including the fertility test that countless people are looking for. (Spoiler: It does not exist.)

MISCONCEPTION: The birth control pill can make you infertile.
FERTILITY FACT: The birth control pill does not make you infertile. In my opinion, it is science's greatest gift to women, with egg freezing in

second place. The pill allows women to safely turn our fertility *on* and *off* while also reducing the risk of many gynecological cancers, such as ovarian and uterine cancer, and diseases, including endometriosis and fibroids. By masking your natural cycle, you may be unaware of a future fertility problem, such as irregular ovulation that is not exposed while on the pill. The pill does not cause irregular ovulation or any underlying cause of infertility; it may simply delay your ability to find out any issues you already have.

MISCONCEPTION: You are able to get pregnant until you hit menopause, which is when your fertility comes to an end.

FERTILITY FACT: "Menses does not equal motherhood," I often tell my patients, meaning that just because you get your period does not mean you can still have a baby. Our fertility ends long before our period ends, unfortunately, because we continue getting our period even when our fertile years are behind us. Most women have a very hard time getting pregnant around 10 years before they go through menopause because the eggs that remain are more often than not unable to result in a viable pregnancy. Menopause is defined as a full year since your last period, so we can only know when you've hit menopause after the fact. It is fair to assume that if your mom went through menopause at 45, your fertility will start to seriously decline around age 35. Pregnancy can still be achieved, however, with your own frozen egg or a donor egg.

MISCONCEPTION: There is only one day each month that you can get pregnant, so if you don't have sex on that day, you will have to wait another month to try.

FERTILITY FACT: There is not one magical day every month during which you can get pregnant, leaving all the other days a "waste," a term I hear from patients who become single-minded about the purpose of intercourse. I have seen couples who think they need to have sex multiple times on that one particular day, which is also not true. Statistically speaking, you are most likely to get pregnant when you have sex the day before you ovulate, but the timing is not like a dart hitting the red bull's-eye. The outer blue, yellow, and green circles on the metaphorical dartboard can still very much lead to pregnancy, so having intercourse five days before or one day after you ovulate is not a waste!

Patients often come in devastated because their partner will be out of town on the *one* day they are *supposed* to have sex, or upset that a flight delay means all bets are off. That is not how it works! While the egg only lives for about 24 hours after it is ovulated, sperm can live for up to five days in the female reproductive tract, so you have wiggle room to get the egg and the sperm to meet, not a strict 24-hour window.

When I was starting out my career as a doctor, I wanted to time getting pregnant so that my third trimester did not conflict with my board exams. If I got pregnant nine or 10 months before my oral fertility board exam in Dallas to become a board-certified fertility specialist, I feared flying in my third trimester, trying to answer the examiner's questions orally while I was distracted by kicking inside of me, or worse, delivering early while I was thousands of miles from home and alone. (But at least surrounded by lots of doctors.) My then-husband and I played it safe, so I thought, by having sex four days before I ovulated. A whole four days before my egg was anywhere in sight of his sperm, so unprotected sex seemed like a safe bet. Lo and behold, I got pregnant, and my due date was April 15, less than a week after the boards! So even a fertility doctor like me can mess up the timing, particularly if you neglect to consider that sperm can stick around for up to five days. Thankfully, I delivered my beautiful baby girl a little early, then flew to Dallas to take my exam nine days postpartum. I am still traumatized thinking about how I forgot to pack a piece of my breast pump, so I was engorged, uncomfortable, and sad to waste my precious milk. All's well that ends well because I ended up buying the missing part and passing the boards, too.

Many patients tell me their timing is off for sex as they show me on a calendar all the days they had sex and the overlap with ovulation. As I said, sperm can live for five days in the female reproductive tract, and an egg lives for around 12 to 24 hours after it is ovulated. So if you are having regular intercourse (one to two times per week), as opposed to during one particular day or hour, your timing is not likely to be off.

MISCONCEPTION: Most menstrual cycles are 28 days, with ovulation on day 14.

FERTILITY FACT: I believed this myth until I was deep into my medical training, so no judgment here! Ovulation timing, meaning when the egg is released, is based on the length of one's menstrual cycle, which varies from person to person and from month to month, so it does not universally occur on day 14. Cycle variability stems from the number of days it takes your body to grow and develop the follicle that holds the egg, which is called the follicular phase of ovulation. Shorter cycles (26 days or less) do this faster. Longer cycles (32 days or more) do this slower. The second half of the cycle, the luteal phase, is 12 to 14 days for all of us, no matter the length of your overall cycle. Ovulation occurs between the two phases. Since it's only the front half of the cycle that varies, the formula for figuring out when you ovulate is subtracting 12 to 14 from the total number of days in your cycle.

If your cycle is 28 days, then you ovulate on (or very close to) day 14. If, however, your cycle is 38 days, then you are mistaken to think that your egg is released on day 14. Were you to have sex on day 14 of a 38-day cycle, the sperm would be long gone by the time your egg shows up at the party. For a 38-day cycle, having sex on or around day 22 is a better bet if you are trying to conceive.

MISCONCEPTION: IVF is risky because it increases your chances of breast or ovarian cancer.

FERTILITY FACT: IVF most absolutely does not increase the likelihood that you will develop cancer. While intuitively we may connect high doses of hormones to cancers that are hormone sensitive, the direct linkage between IVF and cancer is just not there. Women who take fertility hormones to achieve a pregnancy, freeze eggs, or freeze embryos have not proven to be at higher risk for gynecological or breast cancers because of the treatment. There is no definitive evidence of a causal relationship. Taking it a step further, many women who are diagnosed with cancer freeze eggs or embryos before treatment without any increased risk of cancer spread or recurrence. Pregnancy and breastfeeding are protective against breast and gynecological cancers, which may explain why women who have infertility have a higher chance of both breast and ovarian cancer—but it is not because of fertility hormones or treatments.

I was an avid exerciser living a very healthy life. I never smoked and only drank socially, yet I was diagnosed with breast cancer at age 41. Unlucky shit happens, and we do not know why. It sucks. I see all too often how people desperate for answers blame circumstances that have absolutely no bearing on their difficulty conceiving. Myths make their way into the world because we want simple explanations or finger-pointing that makes us feel more in control. IVF does have side effects, such as bloating, transient weight gain, mood fluctuations, and sleep disruption, but an increased risk of cancer is not one of them.

MISCONCEPTION: Sexual position matters when trying to get pregnant. Also, as soon as the deed is done, lay down on your back and lift your legs up in the air at a 90-degree angle or else the sperm will come out!

FERTILITY FACT: Your position during sex and after sex does not matter one bit. While you may prefer a certain position, your fertility does not. Women can get pregnant in almost any position: legs up, legs down, in the bedroom, in the bathroom, or any which way. Sperm does not fall out or find it to be a more arduous journey when ejaculated from behind, on top, or from any particular angle. Within seconds of ejaculation, the sperm is inside the reproductive tract and in the fallopian tubes, before you can even think about your favorite vertical yoga position. Ejaculate may fall out, but sperm is long gone by the time any slides away.

MISCONCEPTION: If you do not have an orgasm during intercourse, you cannot get pregnant. So you better get hot and heavy, not just go through the motions.

FERTILITY FACT: While an orgasm is a plus for pleasure, it is not relevant in terms of achieving a pregnancy. There has long been thought that the contraction of the uterus following an orgasm may help propel sperm to the egg, but that is a falsehood. Many women achieve a pregnancy without experiencing an orgasm. While I do hope you have enjoyable sex and don't lose sight of the fact that intercourse is more than just potential baby-making, there is zero connection between a climax and conception.

MISCONCEPTION: A period is your egg coming out. (If you look closely enough, sometimes you can even see a tiny egg in the blood, right?) That's why you're most fertile during menstruation.

FERTILITY FACT: I do not know what you could be seeing in your blood that has egg-like features, but I do know that it is not one of your eggs (which, incidentally, are so microscopic that they are not visible to the naked eye). About 12 to 14 days before you get your period (mid-cycle), the egg has been ovulated, meaning released from the ovary, is picked up by the fallopian tube, and then given the chance to meet up with the sperm. If it does not connect with sperm and no embryo implants in the uterus, the corpus luteum stops making hormones and the uterine lining (also known as endometrium) sheds over approximately three to five days, which is a period. There's no egg in sight during this time, so you are definitely not most fertile. Anything you see coming out in the blood when you have your period is likely tissue shedding from the uterus.

MISCONCEPTION: You have a 50/50 chance of getting pregnant every month.

FERTILITY FACT: Oh, how I wish people who desired a pregnancy had a 50/50 shot every month, even if it put me out of practice. Like watching my daughter do her homework while she is concurrently watching the Dodgers game on her phone, human reproduction is inefficient and often ineffectual. Most of the eggs a woman ovulates will not make an embryo, let alone a viable pregnancy. Fecundability (the fancy way of saying one's ability to get pregnant each menstrual cycle) is never greater than 15 to 25 percent per menstrual cycle—and that is when we are in our prime reproductive years (think 20s) and have frequent sex in the first few months of trying. The number drops significantly as we age and also the longer we try without achieving a pregnancy.

MISCONCEPTION: Stop thinking about getting pregnant so much! If you just relax both your body and brain, it will happen. Your stress is making it harder for you.

FERTILITY FACT: I wish I could give permission to punch anyone who says this to you or a loved one, but instead I will tell you that infertility is a disease that affects one in six people globally. It is a disease that requires medical treatment, not a condescending and insulting mandate to chill out. Imagine telling a cancer patient, "Maybe you should try a massage, a vacation, meditation, or a potent gummy before considering chemotherapy; it really seems like you are just too stressed out." We would never! Yet with fertility there is often an implication that hardship is psychological, even your own fault, and treatment is called for only after you have adequately worked toward a state of zen. While the hormonal and physical fluctuations associated with stress can impact our health, relaxing is not a panacea for infertility. If you are obsessing about getting pregnant so much that you cannot think about anything else, by all means take a vacation or get a massage in an effort to get into a better headspace, but do not expect this to magically cure your infertility.

MISCONCEPTION: There is a test that measures how fertile you are. Just ask your doctor for "the fertility test."

FERTILITY FACT: There is no test that has anyone walking out of my office knowing if they are fertile, infertile, or somewhere in between. People expect to have blood drawn and then have a finite number spit out of a computer that offers a complete picture of their fertility. That does not exist! While there is data we can gather to measure egg *quantity*, there is a vast difference between quantity and quality. The only test for egg *quality* and one's overall fertility is the ability to conceive a healthy pregnancy.

We can do ovarian reserve testing (antral follicle count and AMH) to assess egg quantity. Sure, more eggs are better when trying to conceive, but the number of eggs you have left may have no bearing on the quality of your eggs. If I test your egg quantity and share the news with you that your reserve is low for your age, that does not mean you are infertile or even close to it. I have, on more than one occasion, had egg freezing patients who knew that their quantity was low based on testing. They mistakenly interpreted that to mean their chances of getting pregnant were significantly reduced, which is not the case when quantity is low but quality is unknown. They proceeded to have unprotected intercourse and get pregnant, which was not their desired outcome, as they were freezing eggs for possible use in the future. There is no way of knowing if eggs—whether plentiful in supply or low in reserve—can become fertilized by sperm and create a healthy pregnancy prior to fertilization. Women with A+ ovarian reserve testing can struggle to conceive, and women with poor ovarian reserve results can get pregnant quickly.

I think it is a great idea to know about your quantity, particularly if you are not intending to try to have a baby for some time. But keep in mind that the data provided is only one piece of your fertility puzzle. There are no markers or tests for ovarian health or egg quality, so we have no idea if an egg will make a viable embryo until it is connected with the sperm and fertilized, at which point we can test the embryo. I will say it until I'm blue in the face: The only true fertility test is the ability to get pregnant. Please be wary of any pop-up clinic that tells you otherwise. They are out there and sometimes are preying on customers' lack of knowledge. I said *customer*, not *patient*, because unfortunately that is often how they perceive and treat those who utilize their offerings.

MISCONCEPTION: Your infertility is, to some extent, in your own hands. **FERTILITY FACT:** Other than having unprotected intercourse at the most opportune time, you cannot control your fertility or possible infertility. You cannot will a pregnancy to happen, and no matter how much you study your cycle timing, cervical mucus, LH surges, and ovulatory symptoms, your underlying diagnosis of infertility will not change. Please do not blame yourself, your body, or your circumstances. Rather than attempting to out-Google your condition or holding yourself to unrealistic, unscientific, and unfair expectations that you must "fix" what is not in your hands to change, I advise you to seek help from a fertility specialist. There are plenty of experts who will suggest you change your diet, consider acupuncture, take a myriad of supplements, and more. I am all for a team approach and there is, in most cases, no downside, but none of these types of strategies are likely to fix the underlying problem alone. Infertility is a medical condition and must be treated as such.

MISCONCEPTION: Frozen embryos are better than frozen eggs, or vice versa. **FERTILITY FACT:** No! One treatment option is not better than the other across the board. I have never cheered for one team over the other universally because the appropriate treatment course varies from person to person and from circumstance to circumstance. In today's political climate, it may also depend on where you live, as recent legislation about reproductive autonomy, particularly embryo freezing, varies substantially state by state. (My patients are primarily based in New York or the tristate area, where I do not currently have significant concerns about embryo freezing.)

Eggs provide autonomy, what I call the ability to take a reproductive pivot, because you maintain maximum flexibility. Embryos give you data about the gametes (egg and sperm) and their potential to create a viable embryo because they can undergo genetic testing but less flexibility because you are locked into the sperm source. In a quality embryology lab, both healthy eggs and embryos will provide patients with excellent options.

If you do not have a partner with whom you are certain you want to have children, I would not create embryos. If you have a partner and both of you want to have children together, I would consider embryo creation. If you want to maintain complete reproductive autonomy, I suggest freezing eggs. I often use my daughters as an example for my patients to understand my refusal to declare egg freezing or embryo freezing superior. I have one daughter who can spike a volleyball with ease while the other can break through defenders to score soccer goals. They each have their own strengths and weaknesses, but one is not better than the other. Embryos provide data in real time, while eggs provide autonomy and can yield data in the future.

Here are some more specific scenarios and my recommendations. I recently had a 32-year-old patient who came to me wanting to freeze embryos with donor sperm. She wanted to be assured that her eggs were good quality, which is information we can gather only once an embryo is created, and she wanted to be a step further down the road to parenthood than freezing eggs, even if that meant using donor sperm. I recommended that she freeze eggs because she might regret being locked into sperm when finding love was still very much a priority for her. Together we made the decision to freeze eggs, not embryos, and when she returned to my office after the pandemic—with the love of her life—we thawed her eggs and then fertilized them with her new husband's sperm. Their beautiful baby girl just turned two and their son is on the way.

MISCONCEPTION: If you are healthy, your ovaries and eggs are probably healthy too. Likewise, a healthy man is likely to have healthy sperm.

FERTILITY FACT: Just like young, healthy women who eat right and exercise can get heart disease and cancer (like me), so too do some such women suffer from early egg loss, infertility, and other reproductive challenges. You can eat well, run marathons, sleep eight hours a night . . . and still get a bum rap in the fertility department. Your outsides do not always reflect your insides, particularly when it comes to your ovaries. Ovarian health is not directly linked to our overall health, so while a healthy version of yourself makes pregnancy safer and reduces risks of complications, it does not guarantee better egg quality or ovarian longevity.

With that being said, obesity can have a negative effect on your reproductive health just as it can negatively impact your overall health. Obesity's impact on fertility is not gender-specific, so there is no playing favorites here in terms of how excessive weight can affect sperm count, motility, morphology, or female reproduction. Women with diabetes and high blood pressure are more likely to have pregnancy complications, including during labor and the postpartum period. Good health overall does not mean you have healthy eggs or will have a seamless pregnancy, but it definitely doesn't hurt.

MISCONCEPTION: Patient stories on the internet are a pretty reliable source of information because most people's fertility challenges and successes are comparable.

FERTILITY FACT: We are individuals (sometimes couples), not machines or carbon copies of one another, so each fertility story is unique. There is not one answer to all of our problems and no social media platform that will give us a definitive answer, particularly when people post misinformation, incomplete information, or a possible misinterpretation of what medical experts have told them. Google, Reddit, Instagram, TikTok, YouTube, or any other online, user-driven source, no matter how compelling or relatable, is not always reliable! By all means, if reading other people's stories online helps you feel less alone, click away. But keep in mind that every case is unique, and arm yourself with information from expert sources as well. The same holds true in your real-life relationships. Although your friends' fertility journeys may seem like a good source of information, what worked for them may not work for you. As much as we may think our bodies are the same, there is endless variety in our physiology and biology, not to mention our circumstances, goals, finances, and more.

MISCONCEPTION: Diet, supplements, and lifestyle changes can change your egg quality.

FERTILITY FACT: I am a huge fan of a healthy diet and lifestyle—for myself, my family, my patients, and for society at large. I am thrilled when patients who are trying to conceive eat more nutrient-dense foods, maintain a fitness regimen, reduce alcohol, or make any other lifestyle changes that we know are good for our overall health. A healthy body provides a more suitable environment for a healthy pregnancy, so as doctors, we encourage our patients to eat the rainbow, destress their lives, and get a good night's sleep. But none of that is a magic bullet that correlates with pregnancy.

Remember that infertility is a disease, one that is not cured by supplements, green juice, the elimination of gluten, or any other dietary modification. (If you have celiac disease, obviously you must continue to eliminate gluten while pregnant.) While some data suggests that anti-inflammatory foods can help scavenge free radicals that would otherwise lead to DNA damage, no dietary or lifestyle changes have been consistently or definitively proven to positively impact one's ability to conceive.

The same goes for acupuncture, massage, and alternative health practices. Plenty of experts may recommend acupuncture, massage, Eastern medicine, or alternative health practices in order to improve egg quality or help an embryo implant, but there have not been definitive studies proving any consistent correlation between such treatments and a higher rate of pregnancy. Women get pregnant during wars, famine, and severe illness. While I do not want anyone's body to be subject to less-than-ideal circumstances, ultimately it comes down to age and genetics. I am all for a healthy lifestyle regardless, and achieving a healthy BMI is a worthwhile goal whether someone is trying to get pregnant or not. If supplements or other treatments help combat your sense of helplessness or offer you strength, solace, or other positive physiological effects, go for it! But I cannot definitively say that any concoction of vitamins, supplements, particular foods, or treatments will move the needle significantly to improve egg or sperm quality, increasing the likelihood of embryo implantation, or changing the outcome of an IVF cycle.

MISCONCEPTION: The hormones from IVF and egg freezing will be disruptive and make you feel out of whack, even a little crazy.

FERTILITY FACT: Most women do just fine with fertility hormones! While the injections can result in bloating, transient weight gain, and changes in sleep patterns, they typically do not make patients crazy or drastically disrupt life. Practically speaking, most people can maintain a normal life while taking them, including working and exercising moderately, albeit not so rigorously that you could risk ovarian torsion. In terms of your schedule, you might need to have several early-morning appointments for blood work and ultrasounds, and then the day of egg retrieval I have my patients stay home, as they may experience post-procedure cramping, bleeding, or fatigue post-anesthesia. (I also tell my patients to refrain from online shopping, as they may be a bit groggy and loopy after anesthesia and regret their purchases!)

My colleague and friend, Dr. Meggie Smith, a reproductive endocrinologist in Tennessee who had her own eggs frozen, reports that she felt better than ever with a little extra estrogen on board, despite the bloating. It was after the retrieval that she suffered most of her symptoms, specifically anxiety and depression. She reminds patients that the finish line in terms of possible side effects is not when the eggs hit ice.

MISCONCEPTION: It could be your fault you had a miscarriage. If only you hadn't . . . [insert any number of scenarios involving physical exertion, medical hypotheses, an unusual turn of events, emotional ailments, and beyond].

FERTILITY FACT: Please listen when I say there is almost nothing you can do to cause a pregnancy to stop progressing. Running, jumping, flying, parachuting, eating the wrong food, or any other activity does not cause a miscarriage. Forgetting to take prenatal vitamins, lifting something heavy, going on a hike, or any other strenuous activity does not cause a miscarriage. Unfortunately, 10 to 20 percent of known pregnancies end in miscarriage, and more than 50 percent of those are a result of pregnancy genetics, meaning the growing fetal tissue is not compatible with life. While there are other reasons miscarriage occurs, it is not your fault and you should not blame yourself. We may feel compelled to point a finger, mostly at ourselves, but there is no finger-pointing when it comes to miscarriage. Find a support system that helps you mourn the loss without blame, most certainly not blame that is directed inward.

MISCONCEPTION: In heterosexual couples, challenges conceiving or infertility are caused by the female partner.

FERTILITY FACT: I will (try to) stay off my soapbox about how the field of medicine has ignored, shortchanged, or blamed women for far too long in numerous areas and instead stick to the data: Nearly one-third of infertility cases are attributed in some way to sperm. All male-factor infertility or infertility due to a combination of both the male and female constitute about half of all cases of infertility, so it is wholly unfair to assume that the female partner in a heterosexual couple is where diagnosis and treatment should begin. Men will produce sperm for most of their life, and it is constantly resupplied, so sperm has a lot more runway than eggs do. However, the quality and quantity of sperm is also compromised by age, genetics, and lifestyle factors. Male infertility is a disease just like female infertility, one that affects at least 10 to 15 percent of the US male population. Examples of male infertility include mechanical obstructions that can result in sperm not being released from the testicles, cases in which testes do not produce sperm at all, or exceptionally low levels of sperm. There are several diagnostic tests that we run to get a better idea of why a couple is not conceiving, but in heterosexual couples we do not—and should not—start with the assumption that it is the female partner alone who needs medical attention.

MISCONCEPTION: If you have unprotected sex for a year and do not get pregnant, you should see a fertility specialist for evaluation.

FERTILITY FACT: Long gone are the days when fertility treatment was recommended (or covered by insurance, for that matter) only after one year of unprotected intercourse. Same-sex couples can have unprotected intercourse for years on end, but the absence of the opposite gamete would thwart their ability to conceive, so that's just one example of how out-of-date that thinking and protocol is. Several lawsuits filed by same-sex couples against their insurance companies helped catalyze the industry to change their coverage. Then, in 2023, the ASRM redefined infertility to account for the inability of same-sex couples to conceive without the presence of opposite gametes. So if someone tells you that you have not tried "long enough," ignore that kind of blanket statement because doctors now make recommendations based on age, partner status, genetic carrier status, presence or absence of both egg and sperm, medical and gynecological history, and overall life plans. We want to help you get ahead of any possible eight balls rather than lose time playing a waiting game.

MISCONCEPTION: If you are nearing mid-30s—not the big, dreaded, fertility-falls-off-a-cliff, life-is-almost-over 4-0—your ability to conceive should be fine.

FERTILITY FACT: I have seen so many patients in their 30s who perceive 40 as a hard and fast cutoff, a doomsday brought closer with each passing menstrual cycle. Yes, it is true that fertility declines with age, but it is not like you are walking on a flat road at 37 and then peering over a deadly cliff a few years later. The rate of egg decline is usually gradual, and that slope of decline actually starts around age 32. The presence of medical conditions (like genetic abnormalities or autoimmune diseases), treatments (chemotherapy, surgery, radiation), or other extenuating circumstances (pelvic trauma or an accident) can unexpectedly turn a steady downhill into a rapid decline, but for most of us it is a more gradual process. Another reason to get the number 40 out of your head as a looming threat is because plenty of people suffer from infertility even before age 35. My recommendation is that anyone experiencing problems—regardless of age—should consider seeing a fertility doctor.

MISCONCEPTION: Freezing your eggs or using your eggs to freeze embryos will push you into menopause earlier because you will lose more eggs.
FERTILITY FACT: Every month we lose a cohort or a group of eggs, and not just the one that is ovulated. Think of it as a "we all go down together" type of situation. Therefore, in an egg or embryo-freezing cycle, all the eggs we take out were going to be lost anyway. It is like the saying "Use it or lose it"—if you do not freeze them, they just disappear. When you are on the pill, pregnant, or breastfeeding, this decline continues, so there is no stopping it.

MISCONCEPTION: If you are not getting pregnant from intercourse, the only treatment option is IVF.
FERTILITY FACT: While IVF is the most frequently prescribed course of treatment, it is by no means the only fertility treatment available to us. We have oral medications, IUI, and donor egg and sperm. Parenthood can be achieved through many different paths, all of which should be discussed with your physician. If you don't want to consider IVF or are reluctant to go that route, have an open dialogue with your doctor about your fears or concerns. Then you can start a discussion about what you do want to consider and what an appropriate course of treatment may be for you.

MISCONCEPTION: Fresh embryo transfers are better than frozen transfers.
FERTILITY FACT: You may prefer fresh veggies over a package of frozen peas layered with ice crystals, but when it comes to embryos, the opposite is true. Frozen embryo transfers are significantly more successful than fresh embryo transfers. They allow a clinic to perform genetic testing of the embryo, which leads to much higher success rates, with fewer embryos

needing to be transferred. When fresh transfers were the standard of care until around 2015, doctors transferred multiple embryos because most were not likely to succeed. Once the technology for embryo freezing was proven, along with the genetic testing it offered, transferring only one embryo became the protocol, with a much greater success rate. Frozen embryo transfers also significantly reduce the risk of developing the big bad wolf of fertility treatment, OHSS. By freezing embryos, the body has the ability to return to its homeostasis, thus decreasing the risk and severity of OHSS.

MISCONCEPTION: If an IVF cycle fails, there is not much more left to try.
FERTILITY FACT: One failed IVF cycle is nothing more than one failed cycle. While it definitely takes an emotional, physical, and financial toll, it does not mean the game is over. My family is obsessed with baseball, so I think of a failed round as strike one, and in this game (which is not a fun one for anyone) there's not a "three strikes and you're out" rule. We can glean information from each failed round of fertility treatment, and it is by no means the end of the journey. I typically tell patients to prepare for a minimum of three rounds, if they can swing that financially, and that the older they are, the more cycles there may need to be. Sometimes just knowing that fertility treatment is a marathon, not a sprint, can make the journey easier.

MISCONCEPTION: It's abundantly clear when I look around at my friends, larger social circles, or my online communities that everyone else has it easier than me. I got dealt the worst hand of all.
FERTILITY FACT: I understand that it can feel like everyone around you is peeing on a stick and seeing the smiley face you long for, but it is simply not true. People overshare when things come easy to them, so you may have a multitude of stories in your face that sound like a fairytale. But one in six adults worldwide will suffer from infertility—and that's not including the challenges that same-sex couples face—so you are very much not alone. Both in-person relationships and online support groups can offer comfort and a sense of community, but not every happily-ever-after anecdote tells the whole story, so take some of what you hear or read with a grain of salt.

MISCONCEPTION: You will gain weight during fertility treatment, and losing it will be exceptionally hard.

FERTILITY FACT: Yes, you will likely gain weight during fertility treatment, but there is no reason it will not come off when you stop taking hormones. I tell patients not to go on the scale during the hormonal injections because, as someone who has battled those numbers my whole life, I know it does not feel good to see any shift upward. I could not even look at the scale when I was pregnant because it was so uncomfortable watching the number creep up, even for the best reason I could hope for. But it is not a real number beyond the process. The hormones cause your ovaries to significantly grow in size. This, as well as the fluid shifts and changes from the hormonal injections, will lead to transient weight gain. *Transient* is the key word there; it will come off when you return to your regular routine, your ovaries return to their usual size, and your fluid shifts calm down.

MISCONCEPTION: Every egg you freeze equals a baby.

FERTILITY FACT: Boy (or girl), do I wish this fertility math added up. As I often say to patients, that math is not "mathing." Unfortunately, most of the eggs we ovulate do not result in a viable pregnancy. As I have said, human reproduction is incredibly inefficient, so each egg is nothing more than the *potential* for a baby. By freezing more eggs at a younger age, the odds are in your favor, but there are no guarantees that even 20 frozen eggs will lead to one viable embryo and pregnancy. If you start out with 20 eggs that were frozen at age 30, we will not know anything about if they are healthy until they are fertilized by sperm. Those eggs might lead to six embryos that go the distance in the embryology lab, or zero. At best, around 50 percent of the advanced embryos will be healthy, which means that in this example, 20 eggs frozen at age 30 might only lead to one or two children. This is just a hypothetical; everyone's numbers are different. There are online calculators that some people turn to for a statistic about one's chances of frozen eggs leading to a live birth. I get it, I love hard and fast numbers too! But these are not definitive, and there are so many factors that we can't account for, including gynecological and medical history, future fertility goals, partner status, and quality of the embryology lab.

MISCONCEPTION: Caffeine and alcohol are off-limits when trying to conceive.

FERTILITY FACT: Not in my opinion! Telephone is a dangerous game, especially if we are talking about some of your favorite things being eliminated. While I am certainly not advocating alcohol use during pregnancy, I am a firm believer in the everything-in-moderation philosophy while trying to conceive. I would not make it the norm to have hourly visits to Starbucks or down a bottle of Chardonnay when trying to get pregnant—or really during any chapter of life—but I also would not give up my morning joe and an occasional glass of wine. Caffeine and alcohol consumed in moderation do not cause infertility, will not have a negative impact on IVF, and will not impact an embryo or egg freezing cycle. While you may be asked to tone down your consumption, it is infrequent that you must completely eliminate either alcohol or caffeine. The US Surgeon General did just issue a warning about risk of cancer due to alcohol consumption. There is no such data showing that alcohol inhibits fertility, but it is clear that alcohol—in any quantity—is not risk-free.

MISCONCEPTION: Smoking and drug use should be reduced, but a pot gummy or a cigarette here and there is not that big of a deal during pregnancy.

FERTILITY FACT: While some habits can be halved or quartered, smoking and drug use need to be cut out completely while pregnant. There is no healthy amount of smoking or toking for those who are pregnant; it's got to go. Smoking is never good for your ovaries, so it should go long before you try to get pregnant. Take this as an opportunity to go cold turkey. As for pot gummies or any form of cannabis, thus far there is limited research on how it impacts fertility, but they should not be consumed during pregnancy.

MISCONCEPTION: You have to get off the pill before you can do a fertility assessment. If you are still on the pill, there is just no point.

FERTILITY FACT: It is true that you cannot accurately assess some of your hormone levels (FSH, Estradiol, progesterone, LH) while on the pill, but you can still see a fertility doctor and do the large majority of tests. It is informative and worthwhile to do an ultrasound, take a detailed medical and gynecologic history, check your egg quantity, check your fallopian tubes, and look at the status of your partner if you have one—all of which can be done if you take oral contraception.

MISCONCEPTION: You need to be off of the pill for three months before you can even try to get pregnant.

FERTILITY FACT: The idea that you need to wait three months to "wash out" the pill from your system is total BS. The hormones do not linger in your body, and there is no increased risk of miscarriage or fetal malformations for women who get pregnant immediately after stopping the birth control pill. Once you stop the pill, you do not need to "see what regular cycles are like" (another phrase I hear all the time) before trying to get pregnant. It astounds me how many of my patients think they do not need birth control during what they perceive as a waiting period. The possibility of getting pregnant immediately after stopping the pill means that if you are not trying to conceive, you need to use another form of birth control. Perhaps this myth took hold because it is true that some women's bodies take a bit of time to adjust to a synthetic-hormone-free existence. For the majority of women, a regular period is back within three months of stopping the pill, and for about 90 percent of women, regular menstrual cycles resume within six months. I suggest documenting the day you stop the pill and when your period resumes so you can understand when you ovulate and plan accordingly—but not because this is a prerequisite for getting pregnant.

MISCONCEPTION: My mom got pregnant practically every time she looked at my dad, so I bet I am going to have an easy time too.

FERTILITY FACT: While we do tend to mimic the reproductive patterns of our mothers, maternal grandmothers, sisters, and aunts, a lot has changed over the years, starting with when we have kids. If, for example, your grandmother had four kids in her 20s and you are kicking things off at 38, it is unlikely her experience is substantively relevant to yours. However, if your mom had her last child at 42 and you are 32, that suggests you should have ample runway left for your ovaries. Infertility, menopause, pregnancy, and any other aspect of women's health should not be shrouded in secrecy, so talk to your female relatives and get armed with information that you can, in turn, pass on to your own children.

MISCONCEPTION: If your periods are so painful and disruptive that you can barely get to work, there's nothing you can do except take over-the-counter painkillers.

FERTILITY FACT: It is not normal to have such debilitating pain that you cannot function. Menstrual cramps that derail you from daily activities must be evaluated by a doctor, as they could be a sign of underlying problems, such as endometriosis, adenomyososis, or other pelvic pathology. There are many ways to treat such discomfort, including but not limited to over-the-counter painkillers. There is no reason to suffer or have your quality of life be inhibited, so I suggest consulting a physician, whether it's your internist or a specialist.

MISCONCEPTION: If your periods are regular, you are in good shape to get pregnant.

FERTILITY FACT: It is a common misconception that pregnancy can be easily achieved as long as a woman is getting her period, all the more so if her period is regular. There are many pieces of the fertility puzzle, and your menstrual cycle is just one of them. For example, you can have regular periods but a fallopian tube blockage, poor quality eggs, a uterus that cannot hold a pregnancy, or other obstacles. If you have regular periods, that's fantastic. But it is not an indication that you will be on the fast track to pregnancy.

MISCONCEPTION: Infertility is defined as not being able to get pregnant after a year of trying.

FERTILITY FACT: The definition of infertility changes based on your age, according to the recently updated guidelines from the ASRM. (Even many OB-GYNs do not realize the definition has changed and incorrectly tell patients to continue to try for longer than they should!) While women who are under 35 are not diagnosed with infertility until they try to conceive for one year, those who are between the ages of 35 to 40 meet the clinical definition after six months of trying. As for women over 40, I recommend heading right into your physician's office to get support and an evaluation.

MISCONCEPTION: My mom had early menopause, so that's what I'm on track for too.

FERTILITY FACT: You might have earlier than typical menopause, that is true, because our reproductive lifespan tends to follow a genetic pattern. However, you are not a carbon copy of your mom, so it is by no means a foregone conclusion. Rather than assuming there is a blueprint for your fertility, I suggest you gather information about your family history so you are informed and can seek care if you discover conditions in your family that may be relevant to you. If your mom had spontaneous menopause at age 42 and you are hoping to get pregnant in your mid-30s, then you should certainly assess your ovarian health in a timely manner. Typically, around 10 years before our mother went through menopause is when we should expect to see a decline in our own egg quality and quantity, so in this example you may very well see a quantifiable change in your egg health around age 32. Remember that family history is relevant but also keep an open mind about how your reproductive path will unfold, particularly if you seek fertility care early.

MISCONCEPTION: Embryos can be tested for autism.

FERTILITY FACT: At this time, embryos can only be reliably tested for chromosome number and known genetic mutations, such as autosomal dominant and recessive conditions like CF or BRCA. Autism is a multifactorial condition, meaning there is not one gene that causes the disease, so currently there is no way to genetically test for it accurately.

MISCONCEPTION: Lubricant is off-limits when trying to get pregnant.

FERTILITY FACT: There are some lubricants that should not be used when trying to conceive because they can limit the sperm's ability to swim and fertilize the egg. Anything with spermicide is a no go. This does not mean lubricants with spermicide are a form of contraception, but they could create an unnecessary obstacle. Instead, hit up your local pharmacy for options like Pre-Seed, Conceive Plus, or any of the other FDA-approved lubricants that are marked as safe for fertility.

MISCONCEPTION: You should stop exercising when trying to get pregnant.
FERTILITY FACT: This blatantly false myth makes my blood boil! As an exercise fanatic who worked out through both of my pregnancies, I know full well how working out is one way many of us stay both physically healthy and mentally sane, especially during what may be a stressful period. How unfair to women to have a myth perpetuating that something we love and need has to be eliminated just when we may need it most! Every pregnancy and person is different, so I suggest speaking with your physician to get a nod of approval about anything in particular for yourself. In general, however, you can most certainly exercise while trying to conceive, going through fertility treatments, and when pregnant. But hear me out, as I am not saying that there are no limitations and all women have carte blanche to take fitness to an extreme. If you are trying to conceive and you exercise so excessively that your period stops, that is a problem. If you are pregnant and suddenly bleeding, stop exercising until you are examined. I also would not recommend trying a new sport while you are pregnant or making your life-long dream of climbing Mount Everest the priority as your belly grows. If you are undergoing fertility treatment, restrictions include jumping, twisting, turning, or running. Also, sports with a risk of abdominal impact or trauma, like horseback riding, skiing, and cycling, should be avoided. For the vast majority of patients who are healthy and active, we typically give a green light to activities like strength training, hiking, Pilates, riding a stationary bike, walking on an incline, and the elliptical. While you are exercising, a reasonable standard to gauge your level of exertion is what we call the talk test. If you would be able to carry on a conversation or sing a song that you are listening to, then you are oxygenated and so is your fetus.

These recommendations may change as a patient's body changes, so as I watch ovaries grow, estrogen levels rise, and pregnancies progress in various ways, I may make modifications to what is advisable. I tell my patients to ask me at every single appointment about their exercise regimen, if they have one, so we can be sure to keep their workouts a healthy part of their life. A cardio junkie may need to take a long stroll in the park at certain points of the IVF process rather than sprinting but can still work up a sweat. While I think it is important to give your body a break from exercise when it needs it (advice I am not too good at heeding myself), lying on the couch eating bonbons is not the only alternative. Find a medical professional who recognizes the importance of exercise in your life and helps you maintain your practice, albeit in a modified fashion.

MISCONCEPTION: Prenatal vitamins will help you get pregnant.

FERTILITY FACT: Prenatal vitamins are not designed to increase your chances of getting pregnant or altering your fertility. They are designed to support a growing pregnancy by supplementing or filling in gaps in your diet that are necessary for healthy fetal development. If you are pregnant and have not been taking prenatal vitamins, do not worry! But I do advise heading to your local pharmacy so you can start now, as folic acid, which prenatal vitamins contain, is important during early pregnancy.

MISCONCEPTION: When trying to conceive, men must wear boxers, not briefs.

FERTILITY FACT: The testicles, which are located outside of the body, are around 3.5 degrees Celsius cooler than average body temperature. This cooler climate benefits sperm production and quality because sperm are not fans of high heat. Tighter underwear, like tighty-whities and briefs theoretically can result in an increase in the temperature sperm is exposed to, but there has been no definitive study answering this question. Boxers versus briefs or any other underwear choice is unlikely to have a negative impact on a man's fertility.

MISCONCEPTION: If you bleed while pregnant, you're probably having a miscarriage.

FERTILITY FACT: While bleeding in pregnancy is incredibly disconcerting, it is very common. In fact, my daughters have heard me take calls from so many pregnant women who are concerned about bleeding that they have memorized my typical counsel: "Some bleeding in pregnancy is so common that we see it in nearly 80 percent of our patients. It does not mean you are losing or have lost the pregnancy. You should take it easy with a modified bed rest for 48 hours, and then see your doctor." By modified bed rest, what I mean is try to stay off your feet or at least limit walking, and refrain from exercise until the bleeding stops. Nothing should go in the vagina (intercourse, tampons, etc.) for at least 48 hours, and if you are on a blood thinner, it is likely you should stop taking it until the bleeding subsides. The majority of bleeding is transient and stops on its own without any intervention, but you should see your doctor to confirm the pregnancy looks OK. Patients with a negative blood type like A- or B- may need to take a medicine called RhoGAM to prevent future pregnancy complications.

MISCONCEPTION: Frozen eggs have an expiration date, so it's best to use them sooner than later.
FERTILITY FACT: Frozen eggs are not the same as refrigerated eggs at the market! A woman's frozen eggs do not have an expiration date, and they are capable of being thawed for use at any point. (I am working under the assumption that the eggs are stored in a high-quality facility, which unfortunately is not always the case.) While your eggs can stay frozen for years, your ability to carry a pregnancy is not indefinite. As we age, so does our obstetrical risk, so at some point you will be too old to put those frozen eggs in your own body. I recommend setting some ballpark dates on your calendar to clarify what you hope to do with your eggs and when, and /or think about if a surrogate might be a suitable option for you.

MISCONCEPTION: I'm too young to think about freezing my eggs! That's for women who are worried their time is running out, not me. Besides, freezing eggs in your 20s is a waste of money.
FERTILITY FACT: If you have not gone through puberty, you are too young. If you are a teenager in good health, I also think you are too young to freeze eggs. If, however, a teenage patient has cancer or a medical condition that will hasten egg decline, egg freezing should be explored. If you are in your 20s, theoretically with time before your fertility declines more

rapidly, I think it is worthwhile to put egg freezing on your radar. (So much so that I am writing this book!) Your eggs are the healthiest, of the highest quality, and the most plentiful that they will ever be right now. Of course, there are numerous factors at play, including one's goals, finances, health, and more. If, for example, you are in your 20s and hope to finish a PhD and become a parent of five, then by all means, it is an excellent time to start safeguarding your fertility potential. If you are in your 20s and do not yet know what your longer-term goals are (and that's OK!), why would you wait until your prime reproductive years have passed to at least start getting educated about the possibility of preserving your eggs? I am seeing more and more women come in to freeze their eggs in their 20s because they got the memo that it is never too early to be empowered, educated, and proactive about their reproductive autonomy. It is my greatest privilege to support women of all ages in owning their fertility.

MISCONCEPTION: I am approaching 40, so I'm too old to freeze my eggs.
FERTILITY FACT: It is true that your chances of yielding a successful pregnancy from such eggs are significantly lower than your 30-year-old counterpart, but nothing is written in stone. In my practice, I frequently counsel women over 42 to hold off on freezing their eggs and consider other options instead, because there is little data showing success. However, if a patient feels strongly about keeping the door open for a biological child— and understands the risks/rewards ratio—then I am open to discussing it. I advise patients about how their age will impact their chances of success, and we talk about the financial and physical risks. When the risks outweigh the possible benefits, I recommend holding off, but there is always a discussion to be had. If the benefits outweigh the risks, then game on!

MISCONCEPTION: Fertility medications can boost your baseline follicle count to yield more eggs.
FERTILITY FACT: It is not true that fertility medications can give you more follicles or eggs. Fertility specialists are not magicians. We cannot make things grow that do not exist in the first place. The stimulatory medications that are administered during a fertility treatment cycle provide hor-

mones for the follicles that are present at the start of a cycle to grow. In other words, whatever is already there will get a boost, but nothing is created out of thin air. If your baseline follicular count is 10, the medications should provide enough juice for all 10 to grow rather than just the one follicle that would grow in a natural cycle. If your baseline follicular count is five, fertility hormones can't trigger 15 to grow. We can only promote the development of what is already there, and by supporting with appropriately dosed stimulation medications, the hope is that more eggs can be retrieved.

MISCONCEPTION: Out-of-balance hormones are why you are having trouble getting pregnant.

FERTILITY FACT: Just fix those hormones, right? Wrong. The blame-the-hormones conversation is one that my patients start up quite often. I am pretty much always happy to chat about estrogen and progesterone, but there is no magic balancing act that leads to pregnancy. Tweaking these hormones will rarely fix your infertility. In the words of my girl Taylor Swift, "Band-Aids don't fix bullet holes." Adding some progesterone or any other hormone you are lacking (the Band-Aids) will not fix the underlying condition causing the imbalance (the bullet holes). To improve your fertility, we've got to address the bullet hole. That is where a fertility evaluation and treatments such as Clomid, letrozole, or IVF come into play. (Speaking of my girl TS, I have on more than one occasion DMed her suggesting she consider freezing her eggs if she hasn't yet, because we should all have options. No response.)

MISCONCEPTION: Inject fertility shots on both sides of your body, or else only the ovary on the side you inject will respond to the stimulation.

FERTILITY FACT: You know the saying in real estate, "Location. Location. Location." With fertility, it's quite the opposite. The location on your abdomen where you administer the injections does not matter one bit so long as you inject yourself somewhere comfortable in your subcutaneous tissue. (That's a technical way of saying the fat tissue that lies right under your skin.) The medication is absorbed through the subcutaneous tissue and goes into the bloodstream, where it reaches both ovaries equally.

PART 3

JUST KEEP SWIMMING

CHAPTER 8

Heartache, Healing, and LFG

PERHAPS YOU PICKED UP THIS BOOK because you are starting to think about becoming a parent one day, or maybe you have been desperately trying to become a parent for years. No matter where you are on the possible path to parenthood, facing adversity at some point in the process is a possibility. This chapter is intended to make you feel less alone when the road gets hard—because you most certainly are not alone. When obstacles seem unconquerable, feelings of shame, guilt, fear, and grief are normal. I have spent decades not just witnessing those dark clouds take hold of thousands of patients but being *in it* with them when they say their self-worth is shattered, their body useless, and their purpose unknown. I validate those feelings because I know how real they are, even as I believe that infertility is not failure; it is a disease and those who face difficulty are not broken, they are just human. We mourn the loss of all kinds of dreams, sometimes for a long time. But we cannot let the pity party go on indefinitely. When the time is right, together we can—and must—embrace an attitude of LFG: Let's f**ing go.

"You Can and You Will"

People often tell me I have the best job. I do. I get to help make families, bring life into the world, provide people with an assurance policy, and help turn dreams into reality. But I also deal with a lot of loss, and I loathe relaying bad news to my patients—but I no longer fear it.

The demise of my marriage when my kids were young followed by my breast cancer diagnosis were the two darkest chapters of my life. I still look back and wonder how I made it through the other side. I can't remember how I got myself out of bed some days, let alone how I took care of two little girls who needed their mommy. There were moments when I got a reprieve from my soul-crushing shock, grief, and fear. (Those were the top three emotions, but trust me, there were plenty of others that knocked me out.) It was in those brief intervals, which started to last slightly longer and longer, that I discovered I was stronger than I even knew. Over time, I also became a more compassionate, optimistic, solution-oriented physician.

Before my divorce and cancer, when I had to tell a patient about a miscarriage, a failed transfer, or any potentially devastating development, I would practically run out of the room right after the words came out of my mouth because I could not take the sadness. Sometimes I want parenthood so badly for my patients that their sadness and my own disappointment blur into a tangled-up bond of sorrow.

Now, as a more mature physician and a woman who has grown from my own set of unexpected circumstances, delivering bad news is not just a dreaded box to check before moving on to my next appointment. I know my patients need to process what I have to tell them, possibly hearing me say the same thing over and over until they can grasp a diagnosis, test results, or an unfortunate outcome. I did not experience fertility issues, so I cannot put myself in my patients' shoes, and they know that. But I can be present in their pain for hours, helping them understand and cope with loss, disappointment, shock, and broken dreams. I recognize the moments when I should be silent and when to speak. "Why me?" or "How the hell did I end up here?" are common cries in my office. I do not have an answer that can diminish the sense of helplessness or self-pity, but I can hold a hand, literally and figuratively, through unbearable pain. Most importantly, I can see the way out of the darkness. So when the time is right, we talk about options and hope. With an open heart, counsel, treatment, empathy, and humanity, I can point us toward glimmers of light.

Not too long ago, seven weeks after implanting a healthy embryo in a patient, we discovered there was no heartbeat.

"I can't do this anymore," the 33-year-old told me, tears pouring down her face. She had already miscarried twice, and the thought of enduring loss for a third time was more than she could take. There are, to be sure, times when I know that patients need a break from the process, or when alternate avenues to parenthood need to be considered.

In this case, I knew my patient needed encouragement, akin to the push I sometimes need at mile 23 of a marathon. I looked at her with compassion and conviction. "You can and you will, if you can find the strength, which I know you have," I told her. "First you will mourn this loss. You will grieve the pregnancy that didn't deliver a healthy baby until you are ready to move forward past the exhaustion and sadness. Then you will try again. I will be right by your side as we find the path that brings you to parenthood."

I have cried with many people who have lost embryos or late-stage fetuses in utero and even babies as newborns. I have watched couples undergo immeasurable amounts of physical, emotional, and financial hardship to create a family. The heartbreak knows no bounds. Time and time again, I marvel that no matter how severe the pain, we have the capacity to tell ourselves, "I can and I will." I am in awe of the fortitude and resilience men and women exhibit, dusting themselves off and getting back up. Sometimes I witness it only after they have taken time to heal, and other times the sheer guts they discover deep within goes hand in hand with their healing.

As much as I appreciate metaphors, I find inspirational phrases to be even more powerful. Some might think they can be trite, but a good quote that sticks with me can be like a parachute if I am crashing hard. The most basic phrase can be what I need to hear to propel me to take another breath, another step, another try. One of my favorite quotes, hanging on the wall in my office, is a Japanese proverb: "Fall down seven times, stand up eight." Be it a fertility journey, a cancer diagnosis, the loss of a loved one, or any other cause of suffering, life is going to knock the shit out of each of us at one point or another. Even when we think we may finally be riding the crest of a good wave, we can still take a plunge that knocks us down. Hit after hit, we must find the strength and courage to take the leap beyond pain. It is a choice that only each one of us can make for ourselves. If the Japanese proverb does not resonate for you, then how about the words of Nemo's buddy Dory from *Finding Nemo*: "Just keep swimming, swimming, swimming."

Patient POV

Ophelia, 34

My struggle with fertility wasn't exactly *my* struggle. When my husband was in his 20s, he was diagnosed with cancer and was told that treatment would not impact his fertility. He decided to bank sperm just in case. I was at a routine gynecology checkup when my doctor suggested we do some fertility testing to be sure everything was OK before we started to try. A few days later, we found out he had no sperm. Zero. I was disappointed but pragmatic and practical. Thankfully he had frozen sperm and insurance coverage for fertility treatment, so I felt privileged and undeterred.

Two rounds of IUI with frozen sperm were unsuccessful. We turned to IVF, which my body responded to well. We got four tested embryos. I couldn't believe my luck that the first implantation was successful. Then, at 12 weeks, after no prior concerns, we discovered the fetus had a birth defect that would not be compatible with life. I had to have a D&C followed by a second urgent surgery because of uterine scarring. It was at that point that I felt the weight of the journey. We were back to square one, which felt like failure. Around six weeks later, I was ready to put the previous trauma in a box and prepped for my next implantation. Again, it worked, and I couldn't believe my luck. At 30 weeks, there was a freak umbilical cord accident that abruptly ended an otherwise unremarkable pregnancy and all our plans. The pain was unimaginable. I delivered the fetus via C-section.

When the time was right, we did another transfer, which failed. That was my lowest point. I felt isolated, stigmatized, paralyzed, and like fertility treatment had consumed my whole life. We started to look at alternative options, but tried for one more round of IVF. To my absolute surprise, it worked. Not only did it work, but my one embryo split into two, and I now have two beautiful identical twin boys!

Looking back, when I think about how I made it through, I think that my gratitude for what I did have, like a healthy husband, rather than focusing on what I didn't have, made a huge difference. Also, my husband once said to me: "If we never have children, this life is more than enough for me." That was totally life-changing for me. We found the joy in being together as a partnership and would frequently remind each other how lucky we were to have each other. I'm also really proud of myself for reaching out to a therapist, which helped both my husband and me. Throughout the process, productivity rather than helplessness made me feel less out of control. While I waited for my uterus to heal, I opted to proceed with another egg retrieval. When I took time off work to recover, I wouldn't let myself sit on the sofa all day. I planned one thing a day that could be as simple as picking up the ingredients to make a nice dinner, going to an exercise class, taking a walk, or listening to a favorite podcast. A lot of friends either didn't understand or didn't want to understand what we were going through, so I retreated from relationships that didn't serve me. I took myself off social media, which instantly removed the comparison to everyone else's seemingly perfect lives. I embraced those who cared deeply and was grateful for their maturity to talk about the hard stuff.

I try not to dwell on the past. My family is complete, and I feel unbelievably lucky. I don't sweat the small stuff, and we laugh a lot in our home. The journey was so difficult, but I get some comfort knowing that any different path would not have ended up with me having our two sons. I can't imagine life without them. We feel like a powerful family unit who can survive anything.

Almost any journey that is worth taking is going to require resilience and grit to make it out the other side in one piece. The ebb and flow of life's wins and losses is normal. You cannot know or fully appreciate joy without also experiencing sorrow. Even sports dynasties that appear invincible must ultimately face defeat. I am a Dodgers fan through and through, so when the Yankees' winning streak in the early 2000s ended, I did not shed tears for them. I might have even gloated in their loss, I admit, all the while reminding myself that winning only feels good because it is partnered with losing (even though it may not feel that way when losses happen, especially to the Yankees). Most paths are not linear, and no straight shot of consistent success lasts indefinitely. As a marathoner, I am always on the lookout for a flat course; without the hills, I could better set myself up to hit my personal record. In truth, however, I know it's when I am forced out of my comfort zone, pushing up and down through the hills and valleys, that the real PRs are set. Maybe it's not the PR reflected in a number that qualifies me for the Boston Marathon, but it is when I learn about life and myself in the most important ways.

There is nothing wrong with having been a fan of Tom Brady and the Patriots in years gone by, or cheering for Mahomes and the Chiefs these days. The Patriots used to win all the time, and the Chiefs are on a current hot streak. If either one is your team, it is safe to say your Sundays were punctuated by a W and a smile. But if you've been rooting for the Browns in recent years? Not so much. In 2017, they went an entire season without winning a single game and clocked the most losses of any NFL team in a 20-year period. Ouch. Losing sucks, but game after game they had to get back up and keep working hard. Their fans, too, or at least the loyal ones, had to also make the choice to continue to cheer. Defeat after defeat, back in the game they go. The ability to persevere in the face of loss is when true grit, character, and determination get the opportunity to blossom.

Now I am not saying that if you, for example, have done 20 IVF cycles with no success, you ought to keep at it if you want your dreams to come true. There will come a point when that is no longer a prudent course of action, a decision that you and your doctor will have to make together. What I am saying is that if you refuse to give up on your dream of becoming a parent, you will make it happen—not necessarily in the way you expect, but one way or another.

Studies out of countries within Europe and Australia, where IVF is largely paid for by the government, show that up to 40 percent of couples exit treatment even when they are likely candidates for success, not because of cost but because they report that they are emotionally exhausted. IVF can take a mighty psychological toll. I get that. That is a valid choice, and a choice that only each individual or couple can make for themselves. I just hope that when people hit bumps on their fertility journey, they can make choices without desperation or hopelessness steering them. If they can uncover their inner strength and push through the pain, they can move forward with courage and resolve, and then pivot to pursue whatever course of action is right for them. That is what it means to fall down seven times and stand up eight.

Patient POV

Johanna, 38

I was around 35 when I went through early menopause. It wasn't until I was 38 that I had the strength to get myself to a fertility doctor and showed up in Dr. Knopman's office to talk about the possibility of using an egg donor. Before I could even get a word out, I started to cry. Both of my great-grandparents on my dad's side had survived the Holocaust. I was raised hearing stories about their resilience, so much so that my goal became passing on that will to survive and fortitude to my children one day. Would using a donor egg be an end to my unique lineage? How would my kids inherit such unimaginable strength if the DNA wasn't there?

Dr. Knopman listened quietly and then told me with no equivocation, "Just as that strength lives within you, it will live within your children one day. You will pass it on in how you raise them. Day after day they will see by your example that when you fall you get back up, that on the hardest of days we find strength and dig deep for courage. I understand how disappointed you are that your children will not share your genetics, but they will share the core of your family values because you will forever be their mother."

It was at that moment that I made peace with using an egg donor. If my great-grandparents could survive Auschwitz, who was I to feel sorry for myself over needing a donor egg because of early menopause? I'm now a mom to a strong-willed two-year-old who is named after my great-grandpa, Morris. Life works in mysterious ways, but I know my ancestors are proud and this was the windy road I was meant to take to parenthood.

Moving Through Grief

Have you ever been asked: If you could have dinner with anyone, dead or alive, who would it be and why? I love that prompt as an icebreaker, and I am pretty sure it was one of the questions I had to answer in my college application. There are a handful of women on my list, some a bit predictable perhaps, including Michelle Obama, Elizabeth Blackwell (the first female doctor), Billie Jean King, and Taylor Swift. There is one more woman whose dinner company would be transformative: Swiss American psychiatrist Elisabeth Kübler-Ross. In her 1969 international bestseller, *On Death and Dying,* Ross was the first to describe the five stages of grief: denial, anger, bargaining, depression, and acceptance. Everyone processes grief differently. The five stages are not linear, nor are they necessarily experienced one at a time. Dr. Kübler-Ross's focus was initially on people suffering from terminal illness, but her framework has since become the most commonly accepted model applied to a wide range of circumstances that involve loss or significant life changes.

After spending decades working with women who experience grief throughout their challenging reproductive journeys, my first question for Dr. Kübler-Ross would be about the role of self-blame in the grief process. I cannot make sense of the internal finger-pointing that I witness among patients who have a genetic disease that is no different than having a gene that sets your height at 5-foot-2-inch or has you wearing glasses at age 10. Time and time again, I see my patients beat themselves up over what they did or did not do; they second-guess if Mr. Wrong could have been Mr. Right; and they condemn their own bodies for failing them. Their mantra often becomes "It's all my fault" when that could not be further from the truth. I would ask Dr. Kübler-Ross if forgiving oneself is necessary to counter the self-blame, or if forgiveness is even more derailing because it lends more credence to the false notion that any component was their fault to begin with. I would want her to help me understand if self-blame is a default mechanism to make sense of the uncontrollable and unexplainable; for some it is even comforting or feels good, which I would like to better understand.

I would seek Dr. Kübler-Ross's insight about how to help people whose infertility leaves them stuck in grief. I think she would tell me that each patient needs to navigate through grief on their own timeline. But when time is of the essence, it is hard for me to let the pain stagnate indefinitely without trying to counter it with action. When I see patients become paralyzed by grief, I attempt to steadily shepherd them along. I am compassionate but also no-nonsense. I am so honest that sometimes I teeter on acting "so casually cruel in the name of being honest," as Taylor Swift sings in my favorite song of hers, "All Too Well." I wear my heart on my sleeve and find it nearly impossible to hold back. Most patients tell me they know there is unfavorable news before I even utter a word. Do not ask me to join you at the blackjack table because I have no game face. I used to think this was a liability and wish I had the self-restraint to not show all my cards all the time. As I have gotten older, I see it as a matter-of-fact part of who I am, an authenticity I can't deny and maybe even a strength. Being honest helps me guide patients even when—especially when—they are struggling with loss. When I think my patients are ready to hear it, I mince no words and say: "LFG. Let's f**ing go."

When I say "LFG," whether to myself or others, I do not mean "Suck it up," nor am I declaring that it's time to stop feeling hard feelings. By LFG, I mean that sometimes it—whatever *it* may be—is damn hard but we have to keep pushing and working toward our goals. Mile 18 might have kicked my ass, but I can make mile 19 a good one. Or at least try. Everything does not happen for a reason; it happens for many reasons. Moving from Plan A to Plan B is not failure. What if Plan B—or C or D—is the one you were meant to have all along? It is just a different version of the story you wrote for yourself. As a divorcée who got remarried, I still have a beautiful family, it's just a blended one. My kids still have a loving dad, and now they have an incredible stepdad too. Whoever said I was guaranteed to find my life partner after my first "I do"? Turns out I nailed it on the second try, and it's even better than I could have imagined. Likewise, in cases of infertility, your road to parenthood may be different than you envisioned, so open up your mind and get ready for what may come your way with an LFG mindset.

Lao Tzu, a Chinese philosopher, said, "If you are depressed, you are living in the past. If you are anxious, you are living in the future. If you are at peace, you are living in the present." Mourning what was to be and overwhelming fear of what is to come can create a paralyzing limbo that I try to help soften up. Part of my job is to help people mourn the past and not fear the future. Science is increasingly at the ready to help, too, as there truly are more paths than ever to parenthood.

Infertility Therapy

An infertility diagnosis can take such a significant psychological toll that one study showed it could be as stressful as a cancer diagnosis. Processing various diagnoses pertaining to fertility and then navigating subsequent care can be stressful, anxiety-provoking, and alienating. Many patients, both individuals and couples, turn to therapists specializing in infertility counseling to help process the grief and loss felt when dreams of achieving parenthood a particular way are shattered, or for support as emotional, logistical, or financial challenges arise. Working closely with a well-trained therapist in the field of fertility can help build coping strategies for what can be a lengthy road.

When I see that a patient is struggling to move past self-blame, guilt, hopelessness, or anger, I may suggest that an infertility counselor join their team of support to ensure comprehensive treatment that enhances both physical and mental well-being. Batya Novick, a therapist whose practice focuses on all aspects of family building, recommends seeking help if you feel isolated, loss of control, depression, excessive uncertainty, or anger. It is normal to have emotional ups and downs, particularly in the wake of fertility obstacles. But, Novick explains, rather than letting anxiety, grief, fear, and loss take over a person's life, such emotions must be identified, processed, and regulated.

An increasing number of women are consulting infertility therapists proactively, often prior to fertility preservation treatment, surrogacy, or adoption. Once treatment begins, infertility counselors, while typically not medical doctors, are well versed in the nuts and bolts of treatment for infertility, so they can be a tremendous resource throughout the process. After delivery, infertility counselors can also help patients with postpartum depression or other concerns.

I recently saw a patient who had done close to 15 IVF cycles, none of which led to a viable pregnancy. She was spending her life savings and was stuck in denial. I assured her there are other roads to parenthood and I wanted to help her get there, but first recommended counseling. After 10 months of working with a licensed mental health therapist specializing in reproduction, she came back to my office ready to move forward with a donor egg.

Another patient of mine was weighed down by rage and disappointment that her husband lacked sperm. Even after they had decided to use donor sperm, she made cutting comments about the embarrassment and resentment she felt for being put in this position. I heard her say to her husband, "I can't believe I have to get pregnant with someone else's child. It shouldn't have to be this way." As if it was her husband's fault that he suffered from azoospermia!

I told her: "I am confident I can help you build a family, but I cannot help you learn how to make peace with using a sperm source other than your loving husband, who has a medical condition that is not his fault." I referred her to an infertility therapist, with whom she worked for many months, and she is now pregnant.

When a patient exhibits signs that they are unable to cope, or it seems that they are stuck on a merry-go-round without any sign that the incessant spinning will stop, it is advisable to seek counseling. Some fertility doctors may prescribe antidepressants or antianxiety meds, but I refer to physicians specializing in mental health instead.

Ups and Downs

Whether you believe in God or not, and whether you are a Christian, Jew, Muslim, Buddhist, Hindu, any other religion, or none at all, maybe you believe in something greater than yourself. I do. Without belief in something higher, life can seem too frightening, vast, and destabilizing. I am a sucker for shooting stars; it started when I was a camper in Maine, lying flat on my back on the grass, making wishes with my best friends all around me. Back then, my wishes were along the lines of "I hope my team wins color war," or "Tomorrow I want to get up on one waterski." These days, my wishes carry more weight.

When I do an embryo transfer, there is a plunger on a syringe that I need to slowly press on in order to gently deposit the embryo(s). I have always thought that pushing it to eject the embryo is like looking at a shooting star in the dark nighttime sky because the embryo and the media that surround it appear as a bright white dot in the uterus. The fact that I have successfully performed more transfers than most doctors across the country has not changed what I'm thinking every time I do one. I take a deep breath, push the plunger, and pray on that shooting star that a pregnancy takes.

Those wishes, as we all know, don't always come true, but I still keep making them. I hope my patients—and all prospective parents—do not give up hope, because one way or another, I am sure they can build a family. By "family" I don't necessarily mean that genetics will be key. A parent is someone who provides support, nurturing, protection, and unconditional love. A family is a collection of individuals who love and care for each other, a crew that stands together through thick and thin with a bond that supersedes all others. If you can sing the words of the song "Stand By Me" together and mean it (at least most of the time!), that is a family.

Remember the movie *Parenthood* with Steve Martin? (Probably not, as it's from 1989.) As a kid I loved that movie, and then my family watched it more recently during Covid lockdown. Steve Martin plays a character named Gil, whose grandma gives him a life lesson that has always stuck with me. Describing to him her first roller coaster ride at 19, she says, "Up, down, up, down. Oh, what a ride! . . . It was just so interesting to me that a ride could make me so frightened, so scared, so sick, so excited, and so thrilled all together!" She compares that riveting experience to the predictability, boredom, even futility of a merry-go-round, which some people prefer. "That just goes around, nothing. I like the roller coaster. You get more out of it."

I love that metaphor. Life—including fertility—can be less like the merry-go-round and more akin to the roller coaster. It can go up, down, have twists, turns, and we don't know what is coming, which can be both awesome and unbearable. We've got to buckle in and hopefully take the ride with someone we trust, someone to scream with, laugh with, and hold us up when the turns are too sharp. That person may be a partner, family member, physician, friend, or just the words on this page as I assure you: You've got this. If you need to hear it from others, then I hope some of the patients I have featured throughout continue to inspire you with their resilience, resourcefulness, and wisdom. You have the capacity to embody and exhibit courage and strength, too. LFG.

CHAPTER 9

Happily Ever Afters

I started this book lamenting that fertility is an unfair-y tale, because a woman's biological clock starts ticking too darn early, which is unfair, limiting, and leaves far too many women with outcomes they did not expect or want. As modern medicine evolves, and as we make deliberate, empowered choices, that unfair-y tale is transforming, giving way to a new paradigm of family building and happily ever afters—the real-life kind that are not perfect but are beautiful and just right. These results can be messy, hard-earned, and end up looking different than anyone could have ever predicted. If there is one thing I have learned with unflinching clarity over the course of my career and life, it is that families are created in all sorts of ways. I have supported thousands of women and men whose fertility journeys turned out nothing like they had hoped or expected, and yet it became part of the story of their life that they can't imagine any differently.

Darkness Before Dawn

Whether you pursue proactive fertility treatment, get pregnant the OG way, or discover that infertility treatment will be part of your plan—or each of those three paths at different times in your life—expect a journey. For some, getting pregnant is more like a walk in the park and for others it is an arduous climb. A night with too much wine and great sex followed a few weeks later by a smiley face or a plus sign on a stick is not the norm, though people for whom this happens sure love to share it! Reaching the goal of parenthood often takes time, strategy, an open mind, and resilience. Again, as the sign inside my office reads, *Fall down seven times, stand up eight.*

In the front of my office building is an iconic piece of art by Robert Indiana that reads HOPE. It stands on the sidewalk like a guard watching over a castle right where patients pass daily, their hearts full of hope as they enter. I urge you: Do not give up hope, because one way or another you can and will build a family if that is what you want. Your end result may look nothing like what you thought when you played house as a child or when you walked down the aisle, but with a never-back-down mindset and modern-day medicine at your disposal, parenthood is possible.

Patient POV

Sue, 44

I was 31 and my fiancé was 39 when we decided to do genetic and fertility testing. We discovered that he had motility issues with his sperm, and it would be challenging to get pregnant on our own. After three unsuccessful rounds of IUI, we turned to IVF. I got pregnant a few times but couldn't stay pregnant. After treating my body like a pin cushion with injections and spending so much money, I was no better off than when we started the process. I couldn't understand why, and because we were doing our treatment at a huge hospital, I couldn't even get a doctor on the phone to talk me through it. We switched to a different clinic that could give me more hand-holding, where I did another three rounds of retrievals, two transfers, and I didn't get pregnant.

We decided to use a surrogate. Ten days before we were scheduled to transfer an embryo, I found out my fiancé was cheating on me. We told the surrogate it was all called off, and at 37 years old I was deep in depression. I had wasted years and feared my window of having a family had closed. *If only I had taken family planning as seriously as I had taken my career, I wouldn't have been in this position,* I scolded myself. *Would I ever even meet someone, let alone become a mom? I'm the one who let this happen.*

I started dating my now-husband, and when things got serious, I told him we should go straight to surrogacy so we didn't waste time. We found a surrogate, got two healthy embryos, and transferred one, but it didn't work. I came to the realization that if having a family was as important to me as I said, I needed to treat it like a job. I ended up quitting my stressful job, meditated every day, and we got three healthy embryos that were even better quality than the round before.

We heard our son's heartbeat inside the surrogate in January 2020, and in June we found out that I was pregnant. We were shocked. I was 16 weeks pregnant when the surrogate delivered our son, and six months later, I gave birth to another boy. Our boys are inseparable best friends. I do not feel any less connected to one child, nor did my inability to give our first son my breast milk for six months make any difference. When I hear about women who beat themselves up over not being able to carry or breastfeed, I want to tell them that it doesn't matter one bit. I believe that the more you cling to what you expect the outcome will be, the harder it is to have a good experience. The universe has a plan. Everything I went through prepared me for motherhood in a way I never could have expected, including how much I love and appreciate every second more than I ever thought I would.

When you feel an overwhelming sense of pain, fear, or paralysis, I think of it as being trapped in a hurt locker. It may feel like you are stuck, but you will emerge, I promise. When you bust that locker door open, you can break free from the hurt and carve your own path toward your desired goals, including parenthood. Years ago, a close friend was stuck deep in the hurt locker after several failed IUI and IVF cycles. When she finally made it to the embryo transfer, she chose to play Florence and the Machine's "Shake It Out" in the exam room. One line that stood out to me, and continues to run through my head every time a loved one, a patient, or I feel trapped in the proverbial hurt locker, is "It's always darkest before the dawn."

This lyric dates back to an English churchman and writer in the 1600s, Thomas Fuller, but it is Florence and the Machine's use of the lyric that sometimes plays on repeat in my head. During my lowest moments I think of it, and I have shared it with many patients who are drowning in a sea of negativity or uncertainty. I do not advise them to spend their life savings doing treatments that carry single-digit success rates, nor am I proposing that for you. I have no crystal ball, and I do not have all the answers. I am simply suggesting that the sunrise has the potential to seemingly come faster and shine brighter when you embrace an LFG attitude, get educated about the options that scientific advancements can offer, open your mind, and abandon unrealistic expectations. When it seems impossible to believe that light will ever surface again, remember: "It's always darkest before the dawn."

Patient POV

Addison, 45

My fiancé and I were out looking for houses, filled with so much optimism and excitement about our future, when the doctor called to tell us I had extremely low egg quality and quantity. He said we should start IVF right away. That was the start of a roller coaster ride that defined the next four years of our life.

After our first three egg retrievals did not lead to any healthy embryos, the doctor suggested I consider donor eggs. We weren't ready to take that path. I needed to surround myself with people who believed in the possibility of my success even more than I did, so I switched to a new doctor who gave me hope. She said, "This can be a numbers game. If you have the emotional, mental, physical, and financial ability to keep going, I think you should." After five more egg retrievals, the doctor called us with the news that we finally got two healthy embryos.

As my transfer date approached, I was waiting for my period but it never came. I took a pregnancy test and was in disbelief that it was positive! My dream came true when I became a mom to a healthy baby boy. We wanted to have another child as quickly as possible, so we ended up transferring the stronger of our two embryos, another boy who ended up completing our family.

I work in a male-dominated industry and didn't want my IVF to be perceived as a distraction, so I had kept it a secret. There came a point, however, when my boss asked me about starting a family, and I ended up telling him I had been through five failed rounds of IVF. From that day on, he became my supporter. It was a huge relief to stop hiding doctor's appointments or cover up my inability to attend important meetings at the last moment when a retrieval was scheduled. I think it's so important for women to share their experience because it gives other women permission to do the same.

On the Horizon

In the years ahead, fertility medicine will continue to evolve in monumental ways. Just as practices that once sounded like they were pulled from the pages of *A Brave New World* are now accepted as norms in fertility medicine, such as genetic testing of embryos, some of the innovations in the works are bound to further transform the field, family-building, and society at large. Venture capitalists and biotech companies may have their own predictions about which developments will be successful, but as a physician, the following are some of the advancements that I find most promising and potentially impactful.

In my opinion, genetics is and will continue to be the fastest-moving and most consequential field in medicine. It is also, arguably, the most ethically fraught. Currently, genetic testing is used to maximize pregnancy rate, minimize miscarriage rate, and prevent known deleterious conditions from being passed on, some which may severely affect a child's well-being or cause death. In cases of IVF, testing enables only the transfer of embryos that lack the undesirable hereditary gene or genes. It can also be used to identify embryos that are more likely to survive in utero and then make healthy babies.

These are developments I have witnessed over the course of my career, and they are life altering. In the years to come, genetic testing may put more information at our fingertips than we even know what to do with.

Genetics has hit the trifecta with reproductive medicine, revolutionizing patient treatment pre-pregnancy, during pregnancy, and post-pregnancy. Before I got pregnant more than 15 years ago, I was tested to find out if I was a carrier for approximately 10 genetic conditions. Now, screening panels exist for more than 400 recessive conditions! Such testing is likely to continue to expand, one day possibly including testing for conditions that are polygenic, like heart disease and diabetes, which are likely caused by multiple genetic variations. This would then open the door even further for possible IVF with embryo biopsy to significantly reduce the chance of babies inheriting serious, sometimes lethal diseases caused by heritable genetic mutations. This may lead to a Pandora's Box and raise questions about when humans are taking it too far. I have a colleague who predicts that parents-to-be who don't test embryos and then use the data to choose the healthiest one will be in the minority and even be putting their future children at a disadvantage, perhaps in our lifetime. My colleague, who is both a physician and an entrepreneur, speculates that patients will one day walk into a fertility clinic with specifications for their embryos far beyond gender and basic health. Does this mean hair and eye color? Height? Intelligence? I am not looking to play God, and it is my hope that the box is guarded by well-trained geneticists, genetic counselors, and bioethicists so that the information we glean is used to improve the health of our children and population.

I suspect that we are also getting closer to cracking the code of unexplained infertility. We still do not know why embryos and uteri that pass all kinds of tests with flying colors sometimes fail to create healthy babies, but that may soon change. I believe that the next 25 years will give birth to (pun sort of intended) a comprehensive infertility genetic panel, testing that would help identify people at risk for conditions that impact fertility, specifically early decline in egg quantity and quality, early menopause, embryo implantation failure, and miscarriage. By identifying who may have a premature decline in egg quantity or quality, or who is likely to have unhealthy sperm, patients could get critical information in their early reproductive years. If they get the heads-up that they are at risk, they could choose to preserve their options of genetic parenthood starting in their 20s or even late teens. In the same way that if someone tests positive for the BRCA gene, they may choose to undergo prophylactic mastectomy or additional screenings, frequently covered by insurance, testing that may one day reveal likely diminished ovarian reserve or premature menopause would give patients options. Patients, for example, could choose to undergo egg freezing, hopefully with insurance coverage, or take other preventative measures to preserve their fertility.

As for making progress in understanding why some healthy embryos do not implant, I believe endometrial receptivity testing with clear clinical utility, as well as analyses of factors in the uterus that prevent implantation will also develop significantly in the near future. Knowing exactly when to time a transfer for everyone—like a personalized timetable—coupled with what medications are needed to allow a uterus to accept the transfer, and the role of the immune system, will be key to making implantation failure a thing of the past.

If I was a gambling woman, which I happen not to be, I would bet the house on the continued growth of genetic testing for embryo health in the next quarter century. It is likely that scientists will have the ability to turn up the dial on the genetics microscope and not only detect whole chromosomal abnormalities and select deletions, duplications, and inversions, but also identify genetic variants within genes that are associated with disease. While this is dependent on researchers' ability to discover and identify the association between complex multifactorial diseases and their genetic culprits, such discoveries would allow for the identification of embryos that carry the deleterious variants responsible for disease. This would put up a big stop sign to passing such variants on to future progeny and be a big step toward eliminating many lethal diseases.

The technology and protocol behind the actual testing of an embryo is also on track for significant progress. Not too long ago, we tested embryos by removing one-sixth to one-third of the embryo in order to analyze five chromosomes with a now-rudimentary technology called FISH. The data was limited, the accuracy just fine, and the embryo often had a hard time recovering after losing a good chunk of itself. Now we can look at all 46 chromosomes (including deletions, duplications, and inversions within a single chromosome) by removing only a few cells from an embryo using a technology that is more sensitive and accurate. It's like we went from driving a VW Beetle to a Ferrari. We not only picked up speed and precision but also safety, as the embryos face lower risk from the new procedure. In the near future, it is possible that rather than examining cells from the embryo itself, the fluid that surrounds it will be the source of information. Like sampling the bath water after a bath, the fluid inside the petri dish containing cell-free DNA will be analyzed, eliminating any invasive testing.

We have not, as of yet, been able to answer the million-dollar questions that women across the globe undergoing egg freezing want answers to: Are my eggs viable? Will the eggs extracted today have the ability to make a healthy embryo in the future? How likely is it that 10, 20, or whatever the number of frozen eggs may be will lead to a healthy baby? Sure, there are statistics and "egg calculators" that can make predictions based on one's age and number of eggs frozen, but how an egg looks under a microscope does not always correlate to how it will function if an embryo is created. Like many situations in life, looks can be deceiving, and there is no way to analyze egg quality at the time of extraction or at any time throughout the process prior to creating an embryo. The true potential of an egg is only revealed once it becomes an embryo. Genetic testing and the ability to analyze the health of an egg does not exist—yet. If, or when, such testing exists, what lies inside the egg, starting with the number of chromosomes but going far beyond that, would be able to be analyzed. If eggs, rather than only embryos, can be tested before fertilization, the calculus of choosing to freeze eggs versus embryos would also shift, as both would be able to provide critical data.

Artificial intelligence will also revolutionize fertility, perhaps shedding light on many of the mysteries that persist in the embryology laboratory. Serial computer images created by AI that can track an embryo's progress will be far superior to what we can see with spot views by the human eye using a microscope. AI will be able to help identify healthy embryos and highlight factors that correlate with IVF success, and will likely help provide the last word on a treatment plan to ensure the best outcome. AI will also be behind automated systems that can track the trip gametes take from the body to the lab and back into the body, and even one day possibly remove humans from performing complex procedures like ICSI, assisted hatching, and embryo biopsy. Recognizing that medicine is imperfect and human error is possible, AI will increasingly be a tool utilized to create automated systems that ensure accuracy.

While the influx of technology into fertility medicine has already improved how many labs operate, even more clinics and labs will jump on the bandwagon in the years to come. Say goodbye to faulty storage tanks inside labs with handwritten notes about patients and their precious gametes, and say hello to automation, electronic witnessing systems, barcodes, computers, and robots. By improving the accuracy, safety, efficiency, and traceability of many tasks in labs, the chance of human error is mitigated and the fidelity of frozen samples is further ensured.

Technological advancements will also continue to give patients more control over their care. From patient portals that are increasingly changing the way information is provided to and accessed by patients, to platforms that offer hand-holding for patients virtually as they self-administer injections or other medication, two-way communication between providers, patients, and third parties will continue to evolve. With automated systems that keep track of what you did and when you did it, patients will find it easier to become active participants in their own care.

While IVF has made incredible advancements in recent years, a procedure called in vitro maturation (IVM) still presented challenges to most embryology teams. With IVF, the production of eggs is stimulated with injections, and then eggs are extracted after reaching maturity in the body. IVM aims to reach the same goal of mature eggs, but with most of the growth and maturity taking place inside the lab, not the body. This eliminates most of the shots and time required in the first half of the cycle. Even in cases when IVM is successful, converting such eggs into high-quality embryos has not yet reached success rates comparable to those achieved with IVF. Change is in the works. Biotech companies are working on mind-blowing developments, such as using stem cells to act as ovarian-like cells, which could ultimately sidestep the need for ovarian stimulation and be a game-changer for coaxing eggs to mature in the lab. Such technology would not only remove the bulk of needles required to undergo IVF, egg freezing, and embryo freezing, but also lower the cost—making fertility treatments more accessible—and decrease the risk of post-op complications.

Also in the works is IVG, in vitro gametogenesis, a technology that uses stem cells to create gametes. Researchers are discovering how to take cells from a person's skin or mouth to create gametes, both eggs and sperm. This technology would eliminate all shots as well as the surgical extraction of eggs. To date, IVG has only been used in rodents, but the possibilities are endless, including removing the need for donor gametes and allowing same-sex couples to each have a genetic contribution to their embryo.

I imagine my grandmothers in the 1930s reading *A Brave New World*, thinking, *Embryos being grown in glass containers? That's ludicrous!* Fast-forward 50 years later and it was accomplished, and then a century later, 2.5 percent of all births in the United States are the result of such technology. As the lines between science fiction and modern-day science blur, I can only imagine the advancements that await my daughters and their children.

From Desert to Oasis

Beyond scientific developments and technological advances (and in some ways, as a result of them), family-building will continue to be reshaped by the increased accessibility and affordability of fertility services. For far too long, the high cost of treatment and limited insurance coverage prevented millions of people from building families how and when they may want to or how and when they may need to. Fertility services were limited to those who had extensive coverage, those with the means to pay out of pocket, and those who could prove their infertility in accordance with insurance companies' parameters. Infertility and pending infertility—often known as aging—were not seen as diseases that should be covered or proactively prevented. Countless patients have essentially been told that they are "not infertile enough" to merit coverage or treatment, and people in same-sex relationships were often unable to qualify for coverage. Such limitations have already begun to change, and although the political landscape can be unpredictable, I believe that coverage for fertility treatment will continue to expand.

Remember when parental leave for fathers or partners was a groundbreaking idea? Then the Family and Medical Leave Act (FMLA) was passed in 1993, and now the ability to take time off to care for a newborn without losing your job seems like a commonsense offering we may even take for granted. Even better than the right to take unpaid leave after the birth of a child thanks to FMLA, about a quarter of American workers, regardless of gender, have access to *paid* parental leave. Likewise, when it comes to fertility benefits, change may come gradually, through legislation or employers, but the wheels are very much in motion for fertility treatment to become increasingly accessible. More and more companies in various sectors will continue to offer fertility benefits to their employees, whether to stay competitive in recruiting or retaining talent, be a family-friendly employer, or ensure inclusivity. When my daughters start looking for jobs in less than a decade, it is a safe bet that in addition to medical and dental insurance, fertility benefits will be a standard offering for all employees.

Advancements in science are only worthwhile if the people they are meant to benefit can access them. As fertility clinics expand across the country, people who live in so-called fertility deserts will increasingly be able to get the support they need. Also, I believe that, politics aside, governments across the globe will become laser focused on numerous aspects of fertility to counter declining population growth. Access, affordability, and advancements will be the hallmarks of the future, and while I cannot wait to be along for the ride, I am most excited by the thought of future generations having previously unheard-of options and reproductive freedoms. The future of fertility medicine is bright.

A Fertile Future

Before most trips I take, I need to go to the pharmacy to buy a fresh package of over-the-counter Dramamine. I have terrible motion sickness, but that does not stop me from going on a boat, riding in a helicopter, crashing in the waves, buckling in for a zipline, climbing up (or down) a mountain, and jumping at the chance to take pretty much any adventure. For me, doing things that make me feel uneasy, uncomfortable, or even scared out of my mind are part and parcel with feeling exhilarated and alive. Ninety-nine percent of the time, it ends up being worth the inclination to vomit. I also love being a role model to my girls, showing them that you can look a challenge in the face, take a deep breath, conquer it, and have fun doing it.

If taking charge of your fertility feels scary, I get it. As you go through your fertility journey, when you are out of your comfort zone, Dramamine is not the answer, but I hope this book can serve as your fertility Dramamine. I wrote this book because I saw a gap in knowledge about the evolving nature of reproductive care and a need for reeducation about our own bodies and modern science. My hope is to inspire millions of women and men to think about and plan for a potentially fertile future, armed with facts and empowered by other people's fertility journeys so they can be aware of the landscape and live unshackled by restrictions, whether biological, sexual, emotional, societal, or otherwise. Fertility treatment, not just infertility treatment, presents an opportunity to take charge of our bodies and our family-building in previously unimaginable ways. Own it.

Acknowledgments

Life is best lived and played as a team sport, including providing top-quality medical care, raising kids, and writing your first book. I am grateful to the lineup that helped me become the doctor, mom, woman, wife, and author I am today, many of whom are my teammates for life.

Sir Issac Newton made famous the notion that we are "standing on the shoulders of giants." Over the course of my career, I have been fortunate to stand on some incredibly knowledgeable, inspirational shoulders. My mentors and teachers in medical school, residency, fellowship, and beyond provided me with the tools to enable patients to build families when and how they want. Your commitment to my education and practice of medicine has helped me become the physician and author I am today. Together, we are steering the next generation to become informed about and invested in their reproductive options.

To my partners, especially Sheeva, with whom I've worked alongside for 13 years: Providing the highest level of care to our patients, each of us ready to sub in when a time-out is needed, is a privilege I never take for granted. Thanks to our exceptional team of CCRM NY nurses, embryologists, patient care coordinators, medical assistants, and support staff, we are able to provide compassionate, transformative care. I cherish our collective work, which is at the core of this book that will now empower people beyond the walls of our clinic to take charge of their fertility. Special shout-out to Blair, Lewis, Jamie Junior, Hunt, Amanda, Suze, Whit, Nellie, and

Chelsea, who show up with their A-game every day, making the world a better place not just for our patients but also for me.

Thank you to my patients, whose courage and resilience leaves me humbled. I treasure partnering with you on your reproductive journeys and particularly appreciate those of you who trusted us with your stories in an effort to inspire and educate others.

Rebecca, you are the MVP of the *Own Your Fertility* team. Without your energy, passion, and incredible way with words, there would be no book. You worked your magic to turn long-winded stories, scientific studies, and incoherent thoughts into something beautiful that can now change lives. Along the way, you went from coauthor to dear friend; thank you for your partnership and friendship.

We have the greatest friends and family anyone could ask for; thank you for listening to us talk about this project endlessly and encouraging us every step of the way. Amanda, you are the ultimate matchmaker and supporter. Gara, Beth, and Jamie, you keep me stylish, fit, and sane. Jennie, Amy, Lisa, and Pilar, you are always ready on deck with counsel and patience. Eric, Jacob, Lily Rae, and Ben, thank you for being the most lovable, committed, understanding pit crew.

Karen Murgolo, you were the first person to believe in our book, our team captain who offered us a playbook and led the huddle every step of the way. Ann Treistman, we are profoundly grateful that you were the one to carry us from kickoff to the finish line with competence and commitment. Your Countryman Press bench is deep with all-star players, including Maya Goldfarb and Devorah Backman; we thank you all.

Many early readers and advisors played an integral role in bringing this project to fruition, including Meggie Smith, Evette Ferguson, Caroline McCaffrey, Mandy Katz-Jaffe, Anna Treat, Cari Lynn, Caroline Vella, Mar Dunn, Katie Witkin, Leyla Blue, and Blaine Heck. Your input, expertise, and candor have been invaluable.

My OG teammates and ride-or-die siblings, Josh and Sam: As a trio, we've had both setbacks and comebacks, and we come through for each other always, no questions asked. My nieces (you too, Carolina), nephew, and stepchildren, all of whom have listened to me talk about puberty, boobs, and periods for way too long: I hope I have inspired you to use your voice to change the world for the better. Pia always tells us that life is not played on our heels. If you want it, get up and go for it.

Mom and Dad, you are my champions. You stand firmly in the ground and continuously provide me with the courage to branch out in a myriad of directions without fear of failure. You instilled in me a kick-ass work ethic, can-do attitude, never-quit mentality, and a directive to leave my mark on the world, all of which have led to this book. I couldn't have done it without you.

Mark, if there were a Hall of Fame for loving, reliable, and invested spouses, you'd have been inducted years ago, but all the more so after your impeccable editing and thoughtful feedback. You're the real deal. (Yup, another contraction!) In the game of life, you block for me selflessly and guide me into the end zone, allowing me to score the winning touchdown. There is nobody else I would want by my side for life.

My beautiful girls, Chewy and Blizz, Char Char and Blake Blake, Chooch and Cuppie: You are my heart and soul. LFG.

Glossary

Owning your fertility starts (and in this case, also ends) with understanding some of the fundamentals pertaining to reproduction. No complicated definitions here, just the basics with a lot of metaphors in the hopes you'll grasp the essentials without falling asleep reading. For my complete glossary, head to DrJaimeKnopman.com.

Aneuploidy: Going back to our Latin roots, *an* means "lacking," so an aneuploidy is an embryo or fetus that lacks the correct number of chromosomes. For humans, 46 chromosomes is the magic number. Whether an aneuploidy is missing or contains an extra chromosome(s), the outcome is almost always the same: a failed IVF transfer, a miscarriage, or a pregnancy that is not compatible with life. Genetic testing called PGT-A can identify aneuploidies in embryos before transfer, which has improved IVF success rates.

Anti-Müllerian Hormone (AMH): If I could only order one blood test for the rest of my career, it would be AMH, which is also known as Müllerian Inhibiting Hormone. Often misinterpreted as the "Am I Fertile?" test, AMH is a tiny hormone with the mighty ability to measure ovarian reserves, guide dosage of fertility hormones, and predict the number of eggs that may be retrieved in an IVF, embryo freezing, or egg freezing cycle. Simply put, the more AMH, the more follicles. The more follicles, the more eggs. No surprise here, AMH decreases with age. Low AMH means low quantity but tells us nothing about the *quality* of eggs, a critical factor in determining fertility, which is why that supposed "Am I Fertile?" test is nonexistent.

Antral Follicle Count (AFC): "How many eggs do I have left?" is one of the most common questions I'm asked by patients. While I can't answer with an exact number, AFC is a diagnostic tool that can help identify the number of small follicles in a woman's ovaries. Using a transvaginal ultrasound, ideally in the early part of the menstrual cycle, this marker of ovarian reserve can help level set both physicians and patients on how many eggs may be retrieved in an egg freezing, embryo freezing, or IVF cycle, and help determine the ideal dose of stimulatory medications needed to rev up the ovaries.

Biochemical Pregnancy: The presence of beta-hCG can confirm that an egg and sperm met, created an embryo, and implanted, but miscarriage can occur before the pregnancy is visualized on an ultrasound. At this early stage of pregnancy, in many cases before a pregnancy is even recognized, the loss is referred to as a biochemical pregnancy. Biochemicals are most commonly the result of abnormal chromosomes in the embryo, and medical intervention is not typically necessary to resolve the failed pregnancy.

Blastocyst: Having achieved the highest stage of embryo development, blastocysts are like balls of several hundred cells that are mature enough to begin what I think of as a division of labor. Along the lines of *I'll do the dishes and you handle the laundry,* a blastocyst divides into the inner cell mass (which may become a baby) and the trophectoderm (which may become the placenta) by day five, six, or seven postfertilization. This division allows for an advanced grading system, inclusive of numbers and letters that correlate with an embryo's future implantation potential, and a trophectoderm biopsy to assess the embryo's chromosomal computation without disturbing the cells that will become the fetus.

Carrier Screening: Just when you thought you knew all of your partner's idiosyncrasies, figured out how to merge finances, and decided which side of the bed you each prefer, it's time to *really* get to know each other by uncovering which genes you each carry. Meeting with a genetics counselor before conception followed by genetic testing is how couples can identify any inheritable recessive genes an individual may carry, if there is an overlap between partners, and what risk of passing any of these genes on to future offspring may be. As excited as you may have been when you and your partner matched on a dating app, finding out that you both match for certain hereditary conditions in carrier screening may not be met with the same joy. Thankfully, modern-day fertility treatments give couples the chance to prevent passing along certain genetic mutations.

Chromosome: Anyone who stores valuable items in a safe may better understand what a chromosome is by thinking of it as the safe of the human body. Chromosomes carry your genetic material, the DNA that makes you you. Human cells typically have 46 chromosomes, 23 of which come from the egg and 23 from the sperm. Getting a bit more technical, there are 22 sets of autosomes (number chromosomes) and one set of sex chromosomes (XY or XX). When the numbers don't add up as they should, the result is almost always incompatible with a healthy pregnancy.

Comprehensive Chromosomal Screening (CCS): There are many ways to analyze an embryo's chromosomes; CCS is one such test that counts the number of chromosomes in the embryo's cells, revealing its ploidy, which is the number of sets of chromosomes. While not as Insta-worthy as a modern-day gender reveal can be, CCS results—hopefully with 46 chromosomes in total—can provide real-time data on the embryo's ability to become a viable and healthy pregnancy.

Corpus Luteum: The goods to maintain an early pregnancy are produced by the corpus luteum. The estrogen and progesterone required to keep the pregnancy kicking before the placenta kicks in are made in the corpus luteum. After a follicle releases an egg, it takes a moment, gets a makeover, and reinvents itself as a corpus luteum. Just like a parent, it goes from housing, protecting, and nurturing the egg to letting it free when it's mature and then being called on for support in the form of the hormones needed to maintain a pregnancy. If a pregnancy is achieved, the hormone of pregnancy (hCG) will signal the corpus luteum that the body still needs it to keep on keeping on. It is not until the pregnancy crosses the eight-week mark that the placenta takes over and the corpus luteum bows (medically termed involution).

Cryopreservation: What once sounded like science fiction—or a term people only heard of in the context of rumors about Walt Disney being frozen after death (not true)—is now a common medical procedure. Cryopreservation is a process of preserving biological function by cooling and storing cells via slow freeze, or through a rapid freezing process called vitrification. In my realm of medicine, this means freezing eggs, sperm, and embryos, thereby maintaining the usability of such cells for future use.

Diminished Ovarian Reserve (DOR): Like the need for reading glasses in midlife, DOR is a normal part of aging as the ovaries' "gas tank" gets closer and closer to empty, meaning viable eggs are running out. Certain tests such as AMH, AFC, and FSH can serve as the flashing light on the body's "odometer" to indicate there's an issue, but unfortunately the egg supply cannot be refueled. When it occurs in younger women, red flags fly and testing is conducted to figure out why. DOR cannot be halted, but the ovaries can be stimulated with hormonal injections to produce multiple eggs in hopes that, for example, frozen eggs can be used down the road.

Egg Maturity: If only eggs took as long to mature as a teenager who can't yet manage her time or who thinks that throwing a party when his parents are out of town will go smoothly. But, alas, eggs mature much more quickly. I think of the follicular phase, which is around day 14 of a cycle, as their teenage growth spurt, and then they are pushed closer to maturity within the follicle by hormones, proteins and growth factors, until they reach a stage called meiosis II or M2, meaning they are ready for fertilization. Fertility doctors obsess over when to schedule the egg retrieval because timing of this procedure is correlated with maturity of the eggs. A high percentage of immature eggs, despite adequate days of ovarian stimulation, can indicate a problem with the IVF protocol or an underlying fertility problem.

Embryo: A cluster of cells formed by an egg and sperm teeming with potential that may one day become a fetus and ultimately a baby. From a single fertilized egg to thousands of cells, embryos are the starting point of human development. Without major assistance from the uterus, nutrients, and blood flow, an embryo cannot progress from cells into a healthy pregnancy.

Embryo Cryopreservation: After an egg and sperm come together to make an embryo, the cluster of cells can be frozen for future use via IVF.

If you're interested in the Team Egg versus Team Embryo debate, which can leave both individuals and couples conflicted, hit up Chapter 3.

Embryo Transfer (ET): Aging myself here, but I will never forget when E.T. (the extraterrestrial) says to Elliot, "I'll be right here," and points to his heart. Gets me every time. Know what else gets me every time? Embryo transfer, also known as ET, which I consider to be the grand finale of what I do in the operating room. In most instances, it is a short and painless procedure that can be performed without anesthesia as the embryo makes its way from the embryology lab into the uterus. A thin catheter is threaded from the cervix into the middle of the uterus, where the embryo is gently deposited. Hopefully, about 10 days later, the pregnancy test will be positive, indicating that the embryo is "home."

Endometriosis (Endo): I love nicknames so much I practically forget the real names of my kids, dogs, or friends. This one is not endearing in the least, but "endo" is the colloquial term for endometriosis, a chronic condition that causes millions of women pain. When a woman suffers from endo, tissue similar to the uterine lining (the endometrium) grows outside of the uterus in places it doesn't belong, like the ovaries, fallopian tubes, and pelvic ligaments. Endo can impact fertility, but there are treatment options.

Endometrium: The tissue that lines the inside of the uterine cavity makes its presence known monthly in the form of your period, but we don't give much thought to this important inner lining until it's pregnancy time. When trying to get and stay pregnant, we need our endometrium to be hospitable to our VIP guest—an embryo—so it can be nourished, protected, and grow into a fetus. An endometrium that is too thin, too thick, scarred, irregularly shaped, or nonreceptive can make achieving a healthy pregnancy challenging.

Estrogen/Estradiol: If you haven't seen *Wicked* you'll have no idea what I'm talking about, but I like to think of estrogen as Glinda and progesterone as Elphaba. Like our favorite witches who each have their role to play, we need both estrogen and progesterone in our bodies to remain in balance. From your heart and brain to your skin and nerves, estrogen—the general term that includes all forms including estradiol, estrone, and estriol—makes you and your organs feel good all around. Estrogen, which is the dominant hormone in the first half of the menstrual cycle, is primarily made by the ovaries, with a little help from fat tissue and the adrenal glands. Thanks to hormone replacement therapy (HRT), estrogen can be delivered in a variety of forms (pill, patch, gels, or creams) to keep the good juices flowing when the body's production slows down or halts during menopause. However, like everything in life, too much of a good thing can become harmful. Estrogen is no different. Balance with progesterone is essential.

Euploid Embryo: My go-to number in the guess-what-number-I'm-thinking-of game with my girls was always four, but when it comes to chromosomes, the euploid (a.k.a. correct) number is 46. Each cell should have 22 pairs of autosomes, one from the egg and one from the sperm, and one pair of sex chromosomes (either XX or XY) for a total of 46. Preimplantation genetic testing for aneuploidy (an embryo that lacks 46 chromosomes) is used to screen embryos to identify the number of chromosomes and subsequently implant only the euploid ones. As our ovaries age, euploidy can be harder to come by.

Fecundability: Probability and statistics were never my thing, but when I became a reproductive endocrinologist, I got a whole new lens through which to view the calculations of chance. Fecundability is the probability of conceiving in a given menstrual cycle. This probability depends on numerous factors, such as age, medical and gynecological history, and lifestyle factors.

Fertility Preservation: This is the umbrella term that refers to freezing reproductive tissue, whether it's sperm, eggs, or embryos. Because a woman's ovaries are on a tight timeline, a proactive approach to fertility preservation can serve as a kind of fountain of youth. Whether for personal or medical reasons, fertility preservation can safeguard one's ability to have children.

Fertilization: After all these years in practice, I still hold my breath every time I check a patient's results to find out how many sperm penetrated eggs to create zygotes, which is the process of fertilization. Embryologists check for the presence of two pronuclei, one from the egg and one from the sperm, indicating that an egg and sperm created an embryo. Affectionately called "fert" to embryologists and fertility doctors, fertilization takes place approximately 18 hours after conventional insemination or ICSI.

Follicle: Among the top five most frequently used words in my vocabulary, follicles are the protector of a woman's most precious commodity: the egg. Think of follicles like the shells that surround the egg you buy in the grocery store, except they are fluid-filled sacs found within the ovary that house the egg and provide key hormones to the developing eggs. When the eggs are mature, like a bird that's ready to leave its nest, the follicle ruptures and out comes the egg. Because follicles are filled with fluid, they can easily be seen on ultrasound, which is how a woman's underlying ovarian reserve can be measured even though eggs themselves are invisible to the human eye.

Follicle-Stimulating Hormone (FSH): Think of FSH like Regina George from *Mean Girls*: If FSH says jump, the other hormones say, "How high?" In other words, FSH is an important hormone made in the brain with a lot of power, starting with controlling the menstrual cycle. It stimulates follicles to develop, setting the stage for the main event: ovulation. FSH values are also helpful when making decisions about the quantity and, in select cases, the quality of eggs. FSH is variable and can fluctuate, but even one high-level reading could suggest that ovarian health is declining, at which point it may be prudent for fertility treatment to become more aggressive.

Gametes: I have always referred to the gametes as "the goods," because eggs and sperm are the keys for the creation of the next generation. Be good to your gametes (as I have said to my daughters many times!), including learning about how they work and how to preserve them. They may turn on you if you don't treat them well.

Gestational Carrier (GC): Sometimes referred to as surrogates, gestational carriers carry and give birth to a baby for others. These are the women who I believe are the closest thing to real-life angels, as they provide a home to someone's embryo and subsequent fetus for nine months. There is typically no genetic linkage between the GC and the developing fetus, as the gamete sources (egg and sperm) are that of the intended parents. Laws vary within states, and a team of healthcare providers, mental health experts, and legal consultants must sign off on this important partnership that is particularly critical for women who are unable to carry a pregnancy.

Human Chorionic Gonadotropin (Beta-hCG): Colloquially referred to as the pregnancy hormone or beta, hCG is produced by an embryo after implantation occurs, so when hCG levels are detected in either the blood or the urine, a pregnancy is confirmed. The presence of hCG signals the corpus luteum to keep producing progesterone and estrogen until at about eight weeks, at which point hormone production, including hCG, comes from the placenta. The level that beta-hCG starts at and its rise in the early weeks, ideally around a 60 percent rise in value every 48 to 72 hours, are an indicator of a pregnancy's healthy progression.

Hysterosalpingogram (HSG): This X-ray uses radiographic dye to show if the fallopian tubes are open and also if the inside of the uterus is normal—talk about a test that kills two birds with one stone! Frequently performed by a radiologist during the follicular phase (first half) of the menstrual cycle, the test will often shed light on the "whodunit?" mystery of infertility causes. Although the HSG can get a bad rap for being painful, for most individuals the discomfort is short-lived, mild, and alleviated by over-the-counter painkillers. In my opinion, all patients who struggle with infertility, no matter how obvious the diagnosis seems, should undergo an HSG.

Intracytoplasmic Sperm Injection (ICSI): Imagine a shy guy who needs a little push from his friends to introduce himself to a girl at a party. When it comes to the IVF party, if you will, the guy is the sperm, the girl is the egg, and ICSI is the procedure that an embryologist uses to push the two together. ICSI is performed in the IVF laboratory, whereby preselected sperm is manually injected into an egg in an effort to achieve fertilization. By getting these two "singles" as close as possible, there is a greater chance that a "match" will be made. ICSI is routinely used in cases of male factor infertility, future embryo genetic testing, surgically extracted sperm, history of poor fertilization in a previous IVF cycle, or previously frozen eggs.

Intrauterine Insemination (IUI): While IUI conjures the visual of a turkey baster and an at-home science experiment, it is actually a medical procedure that requires a sperm lab and a licensed medical practitioner. During an IUI, the ejaculate is centrifuged (fancy way to say spun down), removing the motile sperm from the "riffraff" (white blood cells, debris, dead sperm, and inflammatory cells). Using a speculum and a thin catheter, the A-team sperm can bypass the vagina and the cervix to then be transferred back into the uterus. By putting your best team on the field and giving them a head start, pregnancy rates are increased. IUI is also key for those using donor sperm.

In Vitro Fertilization (IVF): Since its inception in 1978, IVF has "come a long way, baby," to quote the iconic Virginia Slims ad from the decade prior, as it has revolutionized family building. IVF is the main event in the fertility world, in which an egg and sperm are fertilized outside of the body in a laboratory. If an embryo is created, it can be transferred back into the uterus, where it can implant and develop into a pregnancy. IVF is now used around the world for a host of reasons that include tubal disease, ovulatory dysfunction, low sperm count, poor egg quality, genetic diseases, delayed childbearing, single parenthood, same-sex couples, and more.

Karyotype: While the days of using fold-up maps to get from place to place are long gone, getting a "map" of our chromosomes is as relevant as ever. A karyotype is like a map or a screenshot of the chromosomes, which can be used for individuals who are trying to conceive as well as for pregnancies developing in utero or miscarriages. Frequently referred to as the genetic fingerprint, a karyotype provides information on the number, size, and shape of all 46 chromosomes. Abnormalities in the karyotype are often the reason for pregnancy losses and infertility.

Last Menstrual Period (LMP): One of the most common questions asked during fertility treatment is: Date of LMP. Rather than scratching your head trying to figure out what that stands for, you'll now be able to simply check your calendar or any app you may use to track your menstrual cycle. Like the starting line of a race, the LMP marks the beginning of the menstrual cycle, which dictates when fertility treatment can be initiated, when certain fertility diagnostic tests can be run, and sheds light on how long your cycle is by counting the days between cycles.

Oocyte: The big O (no, not that O, the other one!) is the star of the fertility show, the largest cell in the human body. Medically termed the oocyte, the egg is the immature version of the female gamete or germ cell that holds the key to a woman's reproductive future. When it matures, it becomes an ovum, which can come in hot to the fertilization party with 23 chromosomes waiting to meet a sperm (male germ cell) and create an embryo. If fertilization does not occur, the egg disappears. And let me say it just one last time: Women are born with all the oocytes we will ever have; as we age, their quality and quantity decline.

Oocyte Cryopreservation (OC): An egg is an oocyte and cryopreservation is freezing, so this is a fancy way of saying egg freezing. The egg is the largest cell in the body and is filled with water, so it has taken a long time to figure out how not to damage the egg and its sensitive genetic content during the freezing process. Egg freezing remains one of the most difficult procedures for embryologists, but success rates have drastically improved since it was developed in the 1980s.

Ovarian Hyperstimulation Syndrome (OHSS): From bloating and nausea to abdominal discomfort and difficulty breathing, severe dehydration, and even blood clots, OHSS can entail a multitude of side effects ranging from mild to severe following IVF. This condition in response to fertility treatment should never be ignored, as early treatment and attention to factors that increase risk can be the lynchpin to a timely recovery. Pro tip: After egg retrieval, drink approximately 1 to 1.5 liters of electrolyte-rich fluid each day, bulk up on salty protein foods, and monitor your weight and urine output.

Ovarian Reserve: When the little gas icon flashes on my dashboard, I take that as a friendly suggestion to refill at my convenience, but then I end up driving on fumes before I race to a gas station in desperation. Bad idea, and all the more so when it comes to our eggs and ovaries. The ovarian reserve is like the gas gauge for our egg supply. When the egg tank is full, as evidenced by ovarian reserve measurements like AMH and AFC, you have "miles" left on your ovaries and can keep on cruising. When ovarian reserve measurements plummet, it may be time to pull over and see a fertility doctor so you can make important decisions before infertility brings you to a complete stop.

Ovulation: For most women, every month an egg is released from the ovary and picked up by the fallopian tube. It travels down the tube and then, if it comes into contact with sperm—during this most opportune time for that to occur—fertilization can be achieved. If no embryo is formed, then the corpus luteum dissolves and a period occurs.

Polycystic Ovary Syndrome (PCOS): When my girls were little and they had sugar after dinner, all regularly scheduled events like a peaceful bathtime and bedtime went out the window. Like kids with too much sugar, ovaries with PCOS are dysregulated and dysfunctional, resulting in hormones that are out of whack. Symptoms frequently associated with PCOS include irregular ovulation, acne, abnormal hair growth, insulin insensitivity, weight gain, and infertility. Treatment is focused on reinstating a hormonal harmony either with lifestyle modifications or medications. In select cases, IVF is necessary to get the ovaries to settle down in hopes of achieving a pregnancy.

Preimplantation Genetic Testing for Aneuploidy (PGT-A): When this screening test is used to provide the genetic profile of an embryo in regard to chromosome number, it is called PGT-A, with the A standing for aneuploidy. Such testing is one of the reasons IVF has become so successful, because rather than relying on an embryo's morphology (the way it looks under the microscope to the embryologist), its genetic makeup can be confirmed to have the correct number of chromosomes.

Preimplantation Genetic Testing for Monogenic/Single-Gene Testing (PGT-M): This kind of testing on an embryo is used to look for a single gene defect (e.g., cancer mutations, CF, sickle cell). To date, over 1,700 conditions have been approved for PGT-M testing, so if one or both parents carry one of the mutations, dominant or recessive, they can test an embryo and undergo IVF using an embryo that is not affected by the condition to avoid the risk of passing it on to the next generation.

Progesterone (P4): Made by the corpus luteum, progesterone is necessary to maintain a pregnancy. It is responsible for shifting the uterine environment from a proliferative one to a secretory one, which allows an embryo to implant and a pregnancy to grow. However, if estrogen is the good cop, then progesterone is the bad cop because it causes most of the unwelcome symptoms that many women report in the second half of the menstrual cycle, such as bloating, sore breasts, acne, fatigue/sluggishness, weight gain, irritability, headaches, and depression.

Recurrent Pregnancy Loss (RPL): It is Einstein who is credited with saying, "Insanity is doing the same thing over and over and expecting a different outcome." And while I am not sure if this is true, I know that anything bad that happens over and over again will definitely drive you insane. In the case of recurrent pregnancy losses or repeated miscarriages, "the same thing over and over again" will also cause significant devastation and despair. Although the medical literature has not drawn a firm line in the sand for what counts as recurrent pregnancy loss (i.e. two versus three consecutive pregnancy failures?), the treatment always focuses on figuring out why pregnancy is not progressing. As explained in detail in Chapter 5, the most common culprit of RPL is the embryo's genetic profile and IVF with extended culture and genetic testing often breaks the streak of "bad" luck.

Subchorionic Hematoma (SCH): If someone asked a fertility doctor (or our plus-ones who hear us talk on the phone at all hours of the night), "What is the most common call you get from a patient?" The answer is likely, "I am pregnant, bleeding, and freaking out that I am going to lose the pregnancy. What's happening and what should I do?" Bleeding in early pregnancy is incredibly common, so it is not necessarily cause for alarm. The culprit is often a subchorionic hematoma, which is when blood collects between the chorion (the sac that holds the pregnancy) and the uterus, as can happen in the initial weeks of pregnancy. The size and severity of the SCH can vary; some women don't even know they have one until it is seen on a routine ultrasound. Vaginal bleeding is the most common symptom, and cramping can also occur, which can be frightening for women, as these are also possible symptoms of miscarriage. Most SCH will resolve on their own and cause no problems to the fetus.

Bibliography

Introduction

"The Birth of the Biological Clock" (news release). University of St Andrews, January 26, 2010.

Centers for Disease Control and Prevention. *2021 Assisted Reproductive Technology Fertility Clinic and National Summary Report.* US Department of Health and Human Services, 2023.

Kincaid, Ellie. "Why Delaying Parenthood and Having Kids Later Is a Big Deal." *Business Insider,* June 4, 2015.

Peipert, B., Eli Y. Adashi, Alan Penzias, and Tarun Jain. "Global In Vitro Fertilization Utilization: How Does the United States Compare?" *F&S Reports* 4, no. 3 (2023): 326–27.

Society for Assisted Reproductive Technology. *National Summary Report.* SART.

Chapter 1

"About Insurance Coverage." *RESOLVE: The National Infertility Association.*

Amo, Koo, Kim Young-eun, Kim Ji-hye, and Lee Jae-eun. "Egg Freezing Gains Traction as South Korean Women Delay Marriage and Childbirth." *The Chosun Daily (English Edition),* August 22, 2024.

"Average Number of Children Per U.S. Family (Historic)" (infographic). *Population Education,* 2020.

"The Best Companies for Surrogacy Benefits in 2025." *Hatch Fertility,* January 22, 2024.

Binns, Corey. "Why Women Have Fewer Babies." *Live Science,* February 15, 2007.

Blake, Suzanne. "Rich Gen Zers Are Choosing Travel Over Kids." *Newsweek,* June 27, 2024.

Blakely, Ashayla. "Swipe Left: Understanding Its Meaning and Impact on Dating Culture." *DatingNews,* February 26, 2025.

Blumberg, Perri Ormont. "They're DINKs—And They're Taking Over Your Social Media Feed." *Today,* April 23, 2024.

Boyle, Patrick. "Women in Medicine Make Gains, but Obstacles Remain" (news release). *AAMCNews*, July 9, 2024.

Brown, Andrea D., Brady E. Hamilton, Dmitry M. Kissin, and Joyce A. Martin. "Trends in Mean Age of Mothers: United States, 2016–2023." *National Vital Statistics Reports* 74, no. 9 (2025): 1–7.

Bui, Quoctrung, and Claire Cain Miller. "The Age That Women Have Babies: How a Gap Divides America." *The New York Times*, August 4, 2018.

Compton, Julie. "LGBTQ Families Poised For 'Dramatic Growth,' National Survey Finds." *NBC News*, February 19, 2019.

DeRose, Laurie. "Do the More Educated Want Fewer Children?" (blog). *Institute for Family Studies*, January 31, 2024.

Dewan, Pandora. "Canada's Fertility Has Hit a New Low: Why?" *Newsweek*, September 27, 2024.

Dowling, Erin. "New Survey Finds Employers Adding Fertility Benefits to Promote DEI." *Mercer*, May 6, 2021.

"'Dramatic Rise' in Number of Women Freezing Eggs in UK." *The Guardian*, June 20, 2023.

Ewe, Koh, and Rachel Lee. "South Korea Has the World's Lowest Birth Rate, Fertility Clinics Are Booming." *BBC News*, July 10, 2025.

"Fertility Statistics, Statistics Explained, European Union," *Eurostat,* data extracted February 2025 (planned update March 2026).

Friedman, Danielle. "Perk: Facebook, Apple Now Pay Women to Freeze Eggs." *NBC News*, October 14, 2014.

Gilchrist, Karen. "Egg Freezing, IVF, Surrogacy: Fertility Benefits Have Evolved to Become the Ultimate Workplace Perk." *CNBC*, March 14, 2022.

Ginod, Perrine, and Michael H. Dahan. "Embryos as Unborn Children: The Alabama Supreme Court's Ruling and Its Possible Impact for Legal Rulings in Other States." *F&S Reports* 5, no. 2 (2024): 130–31.

Goldberg, Emma. "Your Boss Will Freeze Your Eggs Now." *The New York Times*, June 29, 2024.

Gomez, Ivette, Karen Diep, Mabel Felix, and Alina Salganicoff. *10 Things to Know About Abortion Access Since the Dobbs Decision*. Kaiser Family Foundation (KFF), June 20, 2024.

Ha-yan, Choi. "63% of Babies Born in Korea Last Year Were Firstborns." *Hankyoreh* (English edition), March 27, 2023.

Hays, Jake. "U.S. Adults in Their 20s and 30s Plan to Have Fewer Children Than in the Past." *Pew Research Center*, June 18, 2025.

"Historical Marital Status Tables, Current Population Survey Data." US Census Bureau, released November 7, 2024.

Hodes-Wertz, B., S. Druckenmiller, M. Smith, and N. Noyes. "What Do Reproductive-Age Women Who Undergo Oocyte Cryopreservation Think About the Process as a Means to Preserve Fertility?" *Fertility and Sterility* 100, no. 5 (2013): 1343–49.

"How Effective Is the Birth Control Pill?" *Planned Parenthood*.

"How Has Marriage in the US Changed over Time?" *USAFacts*, updated February 11, 2025.

Hutto, Cara. "57 Companies That Offer Awesome Fertility Benefits" (blog). *InHerSight*, September 24, 2021.

Inhorn, Marcia C. *Motherhood on Ice: The Mating Gap and Why Women Freeze Their Eggs.* New York University Press, 2023.

Jones, Jeffrey M. "LGBTQ+ Identification in U.S. Rises to 9.3%." *Gallup*, February 20, 2025.

Lino, Mark. "The Cost of Raising a Child" (blog). US Department of Agriculture, January 13, 2017.

Martini, A. E., S. Jahandideh, A. Williams, et al. "Trends in Elective Egg Freezing Before and After the COVID-19 Pandemic." *Fertility and Sterility* 116, no. 3 (2021): e220.

"Maven for Employers—Pregnancy, Postpartum, and Back-To-Work Programs." *Maven Clinic.*

Minkin, Rachel, Juliana Menasce Horowitz, and Carolina Aragão. "The Experiences of U.S. Adults Who Don't Have Children." *Pew Research Center*, March 21, 2024.

"More Couples in Korea Are Having Kids Than Japan—But Stop at First Child." *JoongAng Daily*, May 14, 2025.

"New ABA Report Spotlights Rise of Women in the Law" (news release). *American Bar Association*, November 18, 2024.

Nietzel, Michael T. "Women Continue to Outpace Men in College Enrollment and Graduation." *Forbes*, August 7, 2024.

Office of the Chief Actuary. *Table 11—Cohort Life Expectancies at Selected Exact Ages, by Sex and Year of Birth, Actuarial Study No. 120, Life Tables for the United States Social Security Area 1900–2100.* Social Security Administration.

Pergament, Danielle. "Jennifer Aniston Has Nothing to Hide." *Allure*, November 9, 2022.

"Physician Infertility." *American Medical Women's Association.*

Practice Committee of the American Society for Reproductive Medicine. *Definition of Infertility: A Committee Opinion.* American Society for Reproductive Medicine, 2023.

"Progyny Member Guide 2025." *New York University.*

Saito, Jun. "Why Does Japan's Fertility Rate Continue to Fall?" *Japan Center for Economic Research*, June 17, 2025.

Scheckel, Maddy. "Average Cost of College Tuition." *Business Insider*, updated November 12, 2024.

Shachar, Carmel, Lucy Tu, and Bhav Jain. "Fetal Personhood Laws and Their Implications for Health Care." *JAMA* 332, no. 15 (2024): 1231–32.

"Smarter Benefits for Life's Milestones." *Progyny.*

Society for Assisted Reproductive Technology. *National Summary Report.* SART.

"Statistics Explained." *Eurostat* (European Commission).

Stentz, Natalie C., Kent A. Griffith, Elena Perkins, Rochelle DeCastro Jones, and Reshma Jagsi. "Fertility and Childbearing Among American Female Physicians." *Journal of Women's Health* 25, no. 10 (2016): 1059–67.

"Total Fertility Rate in South Korea." *Statista.*

Twenge, Jean M. "How Gen Z Changed Its Views on Gender." *Time*, May 1, 2023.

"Understanding Egg Sharing." *Cofertility.*

United Nations Economic Commission for Europe. *Mean Age of Women at Birth of First Child*. UNECE.

Yanatma, Servet. "Europe's Fertility Crisis: Which Countries Are Having the Most and Fewest Babies?" *Euronews*, September 28, 2024.

Chapter 2

Adamson, G., P. Creighton, J. Mouzon, et al. "How Many Infants Have Been Born with the Help of Assisted Reproductive Technology?" *Fertility and Sterility* 124, no. 1 (2025): 40–50.

American College of Obstetricians and Gynecologists. "Carrier Screening for Genetic Conditions. Committee Opinion No. 691." *Obstetrics & Gynecology* 129, (2017): e41–55. Reaffirmed 2025.

American Society for Reproductive Medicine. *Age and Fertility*. ReproductiveFacts.org, 2012.

"Are Young Patients With Cancer Discussing Fertility Preservation with Physicians?" *The ASCO Post*, November 14, 2024.

Handyside, A. H., E. H. Kontogianni, K. Hardy, and R. M. Winston. "Pregnancies from Biopsied Human Preimplantation Embryos Sexed by Y-Specific DNA Amplification." *Nature* 344, no. 6268 (1990): 768–70.

"Infertility" (fact sheet). *World Health Organization,* May 22, 2024.

"Infertility: Frequently Asked Questions." *Centers for Disease Control and Prevention*, last modified May 15, 2024.

Office of Public Health and Science. "A Timeline of HIV and AIDS." US Department of Health and Human Services.

Practice Committee of the American Society for Reproductive Medicine. *Optimizing Natural Fertility: A Committee Opinion*. American Society for Reproductive Medicine, 2022.

Chapter 3

"2021 Fertility Survey Report." *RESOLVE: The National Infertility Association*, January 2022.

American Society for Reproductive Medicine. "Guidance on the Limits to the Number of Embryos to Transfer: A Committee Opinion." *Fertility and Sterility* 116, no. 3 (2021): 651–54.

Ayoola, Elizabeth. "Lolo Jones Is Freezing Her Eggs at 40 Due to Fears That 'I'm Running Out of Time to Have a Family.'" *Essence*, updated August 5, 2022.

Bartolacci, A., C. Dolci, L. Pagliardini, and E. Papaleo. "Too Many Embryos: A Critical Perspective on a Global Challenge." *Journal of Assisted Reproduction and Genetics* 41, no. 7 (2024): 1821–24.

Chen, Christopher. "Pregnancy After Human Oocyte Cryopreservation." *The Lancet* 327, no. 8486 (1986): 884–86.

Danler, Stephanie. "Emma Roberts Is Ready for a New Life." *Cosmopolitan*, November 11, 2020.

"Does My Company Provide IVF Coverage?" *RADfertility*.

Druckenmiller Cascante, S., J. K. Blakemore, S. Devore, et al. "Fifteen Years of Autologous Oocyte Thaw Outcomes from a Large University-Based Fertility Center." *Fertility and Sterility* 118, no. 1 (2022): 158–66.

Epker, Eva. "Egg-Freezing Demand Is Up 194%, Highlights Opportunity for Employers." *Forbes*, September 23, 2024.

Estudillo, E., Jimenez, A., Bustamante-Nieves, P. E., et al. "Cryopreservation of Gametes and Embryos and Their Molecular Changes." *International Journal of Molecular Sciences* 22, no. 4 (2021): 1864.

Ethics Committee of the American Society for Reproductive Medicine. "Planned Oocyte Cryopreservation to Preserve Future Reproductive Potential: An Ethics Committee Opinion." *Fertility and Sterility* 121, no. 4 (2024): 604–12.

"Fertility Statistics by Age." *Extend Fertility*.

Gook, Debra. "History of Oocyte Cryopreservation." *Reproductive BioMedicine Online* 23, no. 3 (2011): 281–89.

Hutto, Cara. "47 Companies with Awesome Fertility Benefits" (blog). *Reproductive Assistance*, January 27, 2022.

Instituto Bernabeu. "More Than 60,000 Frozen Embryos Abandoned in Spain." *Instituto Bernabeu News*, November 24, 2023.

Johnston, Molly, Giuliana Fuscaldo, Elizabeth Sutton, et al. "Storage Trends, Usage and Disposition Outcomes Following Egg Freezing." *Reproductive BioMedicine Online* 48, no. 4 (2024): 103728.

Kamel, R. "Assisted Reproductive Technology after the Birth of Louise Brown." *Journal of Reproduction & Infertility* 14, no. 3 (2013): 96–109.

Kamerlin, Shina C. L. "In Vitro Fertilization and the Ethics of Frozen Embryos." *EMBO Reports* 25, no. 7 (2024): 2817–18.

Kempster-Roberts, Cassandra. "Fertility Shock—Women Lose over 80% of Eggs by 30." *MadeForMums*.

Kim, Yerin. "Sloane Stephens Wants Every Tennis Player to Have the Choice to Freeze Their Eggs." *POPSUGAR Health*, June 17, 2024.

Kuleshova, Lilia, Luca Gianaroli, M. Cristina Magli, Anna Ferraretti, and Alan Trounson. "Birth Following Vitrification of a Small Number of Human Oocytes: Case Report." *Human Reproduction* 14, no. 12 (1999): 3077–79.

Lampert, Natalie. *The Big Freeze: A Reporter's Personal Journey into the World of Egg Freezing and the Quest to Control Our Fertility*. Ballantine Books, 2024.

LePage v. Center for Reproductive Medicine, P.C., SC-2022-0579, Supreme Court of Alabama, October Term 2023–2024, decided February 16, 2024.

Mercer. "Employers Enhanced Health Benefits in 2024, Adding Coverage for Weight-Loss Medications and IVF Despite Growing Health Costs, Mercer Survey Finds." *Mercer Newsroom*, November 20, 2024.

Miller, Korin. "Halsey Is Freezing Her Eggs at Age 23 Due to Her Endometriosis and Previous Miscarriage." *SELF*, April 27, 2018.

"More Than 100,000 Frozen Embryos Stored." *The Sydney Morning Herald*, February 16, 2006.

"National ART Summary." *Centers for Disease Control and Prevention*, December 10, 2024.

Naylor, Jordan E. "Access and Barriers to Elective Oocyte Cryopreservation in the United States: How Attainable Is Fertility Preservation?" *Drexel University College of Medicine*, March 2023.

Olcay, Orcun, Yagmur Ergun, and Murat Basar. "Historical Roadmap of Preimplantation Genetic Testing from Past to Present; What Is Expected in the Future?" *Journal of Reproductive Medicine Gynaecology & Obstetrics* 8 (2023): 129.

"Olivia Culpo on Fertility 'Fears' Amid Christian McCaffrey Romance," *Us Weekly*, December 1, 2022.

"Ovarian Hyperstimulation Syndrome: Patient Information Sheet." *Royal College of Obstetricians and Gynaecologists*, 2016.

Practice Committee of the American Society for Reproductive Medicine. "Prevention of Moderate and Severe Ovarian Hyperstimulation Syndrome: A Guideline." *Fertility and Sterility* 121, no. 2 (2024): 230–45.

Practice Committees of the American Society for Reproductive Medicine and the Society for Assisted Reproductive Technology. "Mature Oocyte Cryopreservation: A Guideline." *Fertility and Sterility* 99, no. 1 (2013): 37–43.

Practice Committees of the American Society for Reproductive Medicine and the Society of Reproductive Biologists and Technologists. "A Review of Best Practices of Rapid-Cooling Vitrification for Oocytes and Embryos: A Committee Opinion." *Fertility and Sterility* 115, no. 2 (2021): 305–10.

Prakash, Neha. "The Metamorphosis of Mindy Kaling." *Marie Claire*, August 9, 2022.

"Rita Ora Reveals She Froze Her Eggs When in Her 20s." *Women's Health Australia*, November 22, 2017. Originally appeared in *Marie Claire*.

Society for Assisted Reproductive Technology. *National Summary Report*. SART.

Taylor, Rosie. "'We're Running Out of Room for Embryos': Inside IVF's Big Problem." *The Times* (UK), as cited in *The Christian Institute*, August 10, 2023.

Trepanier, Karyn. "A 25-Year-Old TikToker Went Viral for Freezing Her Eggs: What Canadians Should Know." *Yahoo Life Canada (Style)*, April 3, 2023.

Van de Wile, Lucy. *Freezing Fertility: Oocyte Cryopreservation and the Gender Politics of Aging*. New York University Press, 2020.

Chapter 4

Alexander, V. M., J. K. Riley, and E. S. Jungheim. "Recent Trends in Embryo Disposition Choices Made by Patients Following Embryo In Vitro Fertilization." *Journal of Assisted Reproduction and Genetics* 37, no. 11 (2020): 2797–804.

Beebeejaun, Yusuf, Abbeyrahmee Athithan, Timothy P. Copeland, et al. "Risk of Breast Cancer in Women Treated with Ovarian Stimulation Drugs for Infertility: A Systematic Review and Meta-Analysis." *Fertility and Sterility* 116, no. 1 (2021): 198–207.

Cobb, Megan E. "Sofia Vergara: In Vitro Fertilization and the Right Not to Procreate." *Current Issues Blog. Wake Forest Law Review*, March 25, 2021.

"Fertility Drugs and Cancer: A Guideline." *American Society for Reproductive Medicine*, 2024.

"IVF Process." *CCRM Fertility*. Last modified May 20, 2025.

Kirubarajan, A., P. Patel, N. Thangavelu, Y. Sadeghi, et al. "Return Rates and Pregnancy Outcomes after Oocyte Preservation for Planned Fertility Delay: A Systematic Review and Meta-Analysis." *Fertility and Sterility* 122, no. 5 (2024): 902–17.

Klock, Susan C., and Steven R. Lindheim. "Disposition of Unused Cryopreserved Embryos: Opportunities and Liabilities." *Fertility and Sterility* 119, no. 1 (2023): 1–2.

"Making Decisions about Remaining Embryos." *RESOLVE: The National Infertility Association*.

Society for Assisted Reproductive Technology. "Research." *SART: Professionals and Providers— Research and Dataset Publications*.

"State-Specific Surveillance." Centers for Disease Control and Prevention—Assisted Reproductive Technology (ART), archive.

Chapter 5

"1 in 6 People Globally Affected by Infertility: WHO" (news release). *World Health Organization*, April 4, 2023.

"AMA Backs Global Health Experts in Calling Infertility a Disease." *American Medical Association*.

American Association for the Advancement of Science. "The Lancet: Dramatic Declines in Global Fertility Rates Set to Transform Global Population Patterns by 2100." *EurekAlert!*, March 20, 2024.

American Society for Reproductive Medicine. "FAQ About Infertility." *ReproductiveFacts.org*.

American Society for Reproductive Medicine. "Hysterosalpingogram (HSG)." *Reproductive Facts.org*, revised 2023.

American Thyroid Association. "General Information/Press Room." Thyroid.org.

Attia, Daisy. "Chrissy Teigen's IVF Struggles, Babies & Miscarriage." *Infertility Aide*, June 2, 2024.

"Babies: America's First." *American Experience* (PBS).

Bailey, Rachael. "Nicole Kidman's IVF & Surrogacy Journey." *Infertility Aide*, August 20, 2024.

Bloomberg Businessweek. "The High Price of Fertility: Tracking the Global Trade of Human Eggs." *Bloomberg*, December 12, 2024.

Bora, Debashree. "Fertility Services Market Size, Global Trends, Demand, Forecast by 2033." Report Code SRHI1809DR. *Straits Research*, 2025.

Bulletti, C., M. E. Coccia, S. Battistoni, and A. Borini. "Endometriosis and Infertility." *Journal of Assisted Reproduction and Genetics* 27, no. 8 (2010): 441–47.

Colosi, Rosie. "Celine Dion Was One of the First Stars to Share Her Struggles with Infertility." *Today*, June 24, 2024.

Dattani, Saloni. "What Share of Births Involve Assisted Reproductive Technologies Like IVF?" *Our World in Data,* March 4, 2025.

"The Development of Synthetic Hormones." *American Experience* (PBS).

El Hachem, Hiba, Vanessa Crepaux, Pauline May-Panloup, and Pascale Descamps. "Recurrent Pregnancy Loss: Current Perspectives." *International Journal of Women's Health* 9 (2017): 331–45.

"Endometriosis" (news release). *World Health Organization,* March 24, 2023.

"Endometriosis: Causes, Symptoms, Diagnosis & Treatment." Cleveland Clinic, last modified August 2023.

Eskew, Amanda M., and Emily S. Jungheim. "A History of Developments to Improve In Vitro Fertilization." *Missouri Medicine* 114, no. 3 (2017): 156–59.

"Evaluation of the Uterus: Patient Education Fact Sheet." *American Society for Reproductive Medicine Patient Education Committee,* revised 2023.

Falconer, Rebecca. "Read: Tim Walz's Full Speech at the 2024 DNC." *Axios,* August 22, 2024.

Ghobrial, Stefan, Johannes Ott, and John Preston Parry. "An Overview of Postoperative Intraabdominal Adhesions and Their Role on Female Infertility: A Narrative Review." *Journal of Clinical Medicine* 12, no. 6 (2023): 2263.

"Global Cancer Burden Growing, amidst Mounting Need for Services" (news release). *World Health Organization.* February 1, 2024.

"Gregory Pincus (1903–1967)." *American Experience* (PBS).

Gross, Rachel E. "The Female Scientist Who Changed Human Fertility Forever." *BBC Future,* January 6, 2020.

Hines, Ree. "Courtney Cox Opens Up About Fertility Struggles: I Had a Lot of Miscarriages." *Today,* March 22, 2019.

"History of Infertility" (blog). *Colorado Center for Reproductive Medicine,* November 22, 2024.

"How Cancer Treatments Affect Fertility in Women." *American Cancer Society,* last modified January 17, 2025.

"How Many Children Were Conceived Using IVF in 2023?" (blog). *IVF-Hibaby.*

"Hypothyroidism Symptoms in Women: What Do They Look Like?" *GoodRx Health,* September 17, 2024.

"Infertility Stats You Should Know." *Fertility Answers.*

"In What States Is IVF Covered by Insurance? A Comprehensive Guide for HR Leaders." *Maven Clinic,* June 21, 2024.

"IVF History." *IVF-Worldwide.*

"IVF in Denmark." *Fertility Clinics Abroad.*

Kim, Eun Kyung. "Michelle Obama Says She Had Freedom to Use IVF to Create Her Family in DNC Speech." *Yahoo News,* August 21, 2024.

Lunenfeld, Bruno. "Historical Perspectives in Gonadotropin Therapy." *Human Reproduction Update* 10, no. 6 (2004): 453–67.

Maheshwari, A., S. Pandey, E. A. Raja, and A. Shetty. "Is Frozen Embryo Transfer Better for Mothers and Babies? Can Cumulative Meta-Analysis Provide a Definitive Answer?" *Human Reproduction Update* 24, no. 1 (2018): 35–38.

Malizia, Barbara A., Michael R. Hacker, and Alan S. Penzias. "Cumulative Live-Birth Rates after In Vitro Fertilization." *New England Journal of Medicine* 360, no. 3 (2009): 236–43.

Messerly, Megan. "Tammy Duckworth Uses Her IVF Story to Slam Republicans." *Politico (Live Updates)*, August 20, 2024.

Moore, Julia. "Brooke Shields Jokes Fran Drescher 'Shot Me Up' with IVF Treatment Years Ago to Get Pregnant at 2025 SAG Awards (Exclusive)." *People*, February 24, 2025.

Morice, Pierre, Philippe Josset, Christiane Chapron, and Jean-Bernard Dubuisson. "History of Infertility." *Human Reproduction Update* 1, no. 5 (1995): 497–504.

Neighmond, Patti. "Study: Sixth Time May Be Charm for In Vitro." *NPR*, January 21, 2009.

Nikolova, Vania. "133 Stats on 5K Running Races in the US." *RunRepeat.com*, November 3, 2023.

Ombelet, Willem, and Jan Van Robays. "Artificial Insemination History: Hurdles and Milestones." *Facts, Views & Vision in ObGyn* 7, no. 2 (2015): 137–43.

Petter, Olivia. "'It's So Tough Emotionally': Khloe Kardashian Opens Up about Fertility Struggles as She Tries for Second Child." *The Independent*, March 20, 2021.

Practice Committee of the American Society for Reproductive Medicine. "Endometriosis and Infertility: A Committee Opinion." *Fertility and Sterility* 98, no. 3 (2012): 591–98.

Practice Committee of the American Society for Reproductive Medicine. "Evaluation and Treatment of Recurrent Pregnancy Loss: A Committee Opinion." *Fertility and Sterility* 98, no. 5 (2012): 1103–11.

Practice Committee of the American Society for Reproductive Medicine. "Evidence-Based Treatments for Couples with Unexplained Infertility: A Guideline." *Fertility and Sterility* 113, no. 3 (2020): 605–22.

Practice Committee of the American Society for Reproductive Medicine. "Fertility Evaluation of Infertile Women: A Committee Opinion." *Fertility and Sterility* 116, no. 5 (2021): 1255–65.

Practice Committee of the American Society for Reproductive Medicine. "Fertility Preservation in Patients Undergoing Gonadotoxic Therapy or Gonadectomy: A Committee Opinion." *Fertility and Sterility* 110, no. 3 (2018): 380–86.

Practice Committee of the American Society for Reproductive Medicine. "The Role of Immunotherapy in In Vitro Fertilization: A Guideline." *Fertility and Sterility* 107, no. 3 (2017): 527–36.

Practice Committee of the American Society for Reproductive Medicine. "Standard Embryo Transfer Protocol Template: A Committee Opinion." *Fertility and Sterility* 107, no. 6 (2017): 1399–1406.

Practice Committee of the American Society for Reproductive Medicine. "Subclinical Hypothyroidism in the Infertile Female Population: A Guideline." *Fertility and Sterility* 114, no. 1 (2020): 46–52.

Practice Committee of the American Society for Reproductive Medicine. "Tobacco or Marijuana Use and Infertility: A Committee Opinion." *Fertility and Sterility* 121, no. 5 (2023): 1011–17.

Practice Committees of the American Society for Reproductive Medicine and the Society for Reproductive Endocrinology and Infertility. "Use of Exogenous Gonadotropins for Ovulation Induction in Anovulatory Women: A Committee Opinion." *Fertility and Sterility* 115, no. 4 (2021): 957–68.

Raper, Vivienne. "World Health Organisation Recognises Infertility as a Disease." *IVF-Worldwide*, November 30, 2009.

Refaey, Mohamed, Hidayatullah Hamidi, Sicaja M., et al. "Uterus." Radiopaedia.org, updated June 15, 2025.

Sharma, R. S., R. Saxena, and R. Singh. "Infertility and Assisted Reproduction: A Historical & Modern Scientific Perspective." *Indian Journal of Medical Research* 148, Suppl. 1 (2018): S10–S14.

Slater, Georgia. "Kourtney Kardashian Underwent '5 Failed IVF Cycles and 3 Retrievals' Before Getting Pregnant with Son Rocky." *People*, May 27, 2024.

Smith, Andrew, Kate Tilling, Scott M. Nelson, and Debbie A. Lawlor. "Live-Birth Rate Associated with Repeat In Vitro Fertilisation Treatment Cycles." *JAMA* 314, no. 24 (2015): 2654–62.

Smith, Stephen. "Infertility Timeline." *The Fertility Race*. American RadioWorks, September 1999.

Sole, Elise. "Tyra Banks Says IVF Made Her Feel Inadequate," *Today*, April 14, 2025.

Thompson, Charis. "IVF Global Histories, USA: Between Rock and a Marketplace." *Reproductive Biomedicine & Society Online* 2 (2016): 128–35.

"Unexplained Infertility: Tests, Diagnosis & Treatment." Cleveland Clinic, last modified June 7, 2022.

Union, Gabrielle. "The Hard Truth About My Surrogacy Journey." *Time*, September 10, 2021.

"U.S. Fertility Clinics Market to 2028: Increasing Awareness of Fertility Treatments Drives Growth" (news release). *Yahoo Finance*, updated July 12, 2023.

"U.S. IVF Usage Increases in 2023, Leads to Over 95,000 Babies Born." (news release). *American Society for Reproductive Medicine*, April 23, 2025.

Wilcox, Allen J., Charles R. Weinberg, John F. O'Connor, et al. "Incidence of Early Loss of Pregnancy." *New England Journal of Medicine* 319, no. 4 (1988): 189–94.

Wolfe, Dani. "How Much Does the Uterus Grow in Pregnancy?" *The Bump*, March 28, 2024.

Zargar, M., S. Dehdashti, M. Najafian, and P. M. Choghakabodi. "Pregnancy Outcomes Following In Vitro Fertilization Using Fresh or Frozen Embryo Transfer." *JBRA Assisted Reproduction* 25, no. 4 (2021): 570–74.

Chapter 6

"4 Famous Gay Dads Who Used Donor Eggs to Grow Their Families." *MyEggBank*, June 19, 2024.

"7 Facts with Statistics about Single Mothers By Choice." *Cryos International Sperm Bank*, February 22, 2021.

"Age Restrictions in Japan: Drinking, Smoking, Voting & More." *Japan Living Guide*, April 3, 2023; updated May 13, 2025.

Aime, Maggie. "How Much Do Egg Donors Get Paid?" *GoodRx*, December 3, 2024.

Alaska Division of Motor Vehicles. "Your First Alaska Driver's License." *Alaska.gov*.

American Society for Reproductive Medicine (ASRM). "Gamete and Embryo Donation Guidance." *Fertility and Sterility* 122, no. 5 (2024): 799–813.

American Society for Reproductive Medicine. "Informing Offspring of Their Conception by Gamete or Embryo Donation: An Ethics Committee Opinion." *Fertility and Sterility* 109, no. 4 (2018): 601–5.

"Anonymous Donations: Different Rules around the World." *Sensitive Matters*, September 6, 2023.

Arató, László. "Assisted Reproduction in Hungary Has a Success Rate of 2%." *European Data Journalism Network*, February 15, 2022.

"Argentina Voting Age Lowered from 18 to 16." *BBC News*, November 1, 2012.

Arkansas Department of Finance and Administration. "Learner's and Intermediate License." *Arkansas.gov*.

Arocho, R., E. B. Lozano, and C. T. Halpern. "Estimates of Donated Sperm Use in the United States: National Survey of Family Growth 1995–2017." *Fertility and Sterility* 112, no. 4 (2019): 718–23.

"Average Success Rates for Egg Donation." *The Donor Solution*.

Bittner, Chantal. "Egg Donation: A Victory for Reproductive Justice or Another Handmaid's Tale?" *Petrie-Flom Center for Health Law Policy, Biotechnology, and Bioethics at Harvard Law School*, February 4, 2025.

Brandao, P., and N. Garrido. "Commercial Surrogacy: An Overview." *Revista Brasileira de Ginecologia e Obstetrícia* 44, no. 12 (2022): 1141–58.

Bruton, Paige, and Mizy Clifton. "White US Egg Donors Paid Up to Eight Times More Than Black Donors, Study Finds." *Semafor*, September 2, 2024.

Bubola, Emma. "Italy Bans Surrogacy Abroad, a Blow to Gay and Infertile Couples." *The New York Times*, October 16, 2024.

Bustillo, M., J. E. Buster, and S. W. Cohen. "Delivery of a Healthy Infant Following Nonsurgical Ovum Transfer." *JAMA* 251, no. 7 (1984): 889.

Cahn, Naomi, and Jennifer Collins. "Fully Informed Consent for Prospective Egg Donors." *AMA Journal of Ethics* 16, no. 1 (2014): 49–56.

"Celebrities Who Have Used Egg Donation to Grow Their Families." *Chosen Egg Bank*, November 1, 2024.

"Celebrities Who Used an Egg Donor/Surrogate." *Elevate Baby*, September 1, 2022.

"Chapter 8: Donation." *Fertility and Sterility* 87, no. 4 (Supplement 1, 2007): S28–S32.

Chhagani, Neelam. "Countries Where Surrogacy Is Legal." *IVF Conceptions*.

Cohen, G., T. Coan, M. Ottey, and C. Boyd. "Sperm Donor Anonymity and Compensation: An Experiment with American Sperm Donors." *Journal of Law and the Biosciences* 3, no. 3 (2016): 468–88.

"A Complete Legal Guide to Sperm Donor Laws in Australia." *Australian Family Lawyers*.

Wiginton, Keri. "Cycle Syncing: What It Is and How It Works." *WebMD*, August 11, 2024.

Department of Health Research, Ministry of Health and Family Welfare, Government of India. *Final Rules for Assisted Reproductive Technology (ART) and Surrogacy*. National ART & Surrogacy Portal.

"Donating Eggs FAQs." *London Egg Bank*.

Dubois, B., H. Naveed, K. Nietsch, et al. "A Systematic Review of Reproductive Technologies for Shared Conception in Same-Sex Female Couples." *Fertility and Sterility* 122, no. 5 (2024): 774–82.

"Egg Donation, Embryo Donation, Surrogacy." *Leopoldina* (German National Academy of Sciences).

"Egg Donation Laws by Country—A Comprehensive Guide." *Eggdonationfriends*, June 2, 2025.

Ethics Committee of the American Society for Reproductive Medicine. "Consideration of the Gestational Carrier: An Ethics Committee Opinion." *Fertility and Sterility* 119, no. 4 (2023): 583–88.

Ethics Committee of the American Society for Reproductive Medicine. "Defining Embryo Donation: An Ethics Committee Opinion." *American Society for Reproductive Medicine* 119, no. 6. (2023): 944–46.

Ethics Committee of the American Society for Reproductive Medicine. "Interests, Obligations, and Rights in Gamete and Embryo Donation: An Ethics Committee Opinion." *Fertility and Sterility* 99, no. 1 (2013): 5–10.

Ethics and Practice Committees of the American Society for Reproductive Medicine. "Updated Terminology for Gamete and Embryo Donors: Directed (Identified) to Replace 'Known' and Nonidentified to Replace 'Anonymous': A Committee Opinion." *Fertility and Sterility* 101, no. 3 (2014): 743–46.

European Society of Human Reproduction and Embryology. "Europe Moves towards Complete Statutory Regulation of ART" (news release). *EurekAlert!*, February 5, 2020.

Executive Office of the Governor, Communications Division. "Gov. Whitmer Signs Bills Decriminalizing Surrogacy and Protecting IVF" (news release). *Michigan Governor's Office*, April 1, 2024.

"The First Contested Surrogacy Case: The Story of Baby M" (blog). *Family Source Consultants*, October 21, 2021.

"Fertility Laws Mexico." *LIV Fertility Center.*

"Fertility Law: Germany." *The Fertility Talk*, last modified August 23, 2020.

"Germany Plans to Legalize Egg Donation." *The Surrogacy Law Center*, July 12, 2024.

Government of Alberta. "Steps to Getting a Driver's Licence." *Alberta.ca*, last modified April 1, 2023.

Groll, Daniel. "'Who Am I?': The Ethics of Sperm and Egg Donation." *Center for Bioethics, University of Minnesota*, October 11, 2021.

Groskop, Viv. "What Is the Truth Behind Sarah Jessica Parker's Use of a Surrogate?" *The Guardian*, April 30, 2009.

"The Growing Use of Donor Sperm in the UK." *Surrogacy Lawyer.*

Hanawalt, Zara. "Celebrities Who Have Opened Up About Using Donor Eggs." *Rescripted*, April 2, 2024.

Hashiloni-Dolev, Yael, and Nitzan Rimon-Zarfaty. "Egg Freezing in Israel: Legal Framework and Women's Viewpoints." *Petrie-Flom Center for Health Law Policy, Biotechnology, and Bioethics at Harvard Law School*, September 13, 2023.

"HFEA: UK Fertility Regulator." *Human Fertilisation and Embryology Authority (HFEA).*

"History of Surrogacy" (blog). *Creative Family Connections.*

"The History of Surrogacy: A Legal Timeline" (blog). *Worldwide Surrogacy Specialists*, April 12, 2021.

Hochman, Anndee. "Choosing Single Parenthood in a Pandemic." *WebMD.*

"How Much Do Different European Countries Pay Egg Donors?" *IVF Babble,* December 2024.

Huang, Zheping. "Single Women in China Turn to Egg Freezing as Social Pressures Mount." *NBC News,* October 5, 2022.

Instituto Bernabeu. "Legislation in Spain and Europe on Assisted Reproduction." Instituto Bernabeu – Assisted Reproduction.

"IVF in Europe: Laws and Restrictions." *ProLife Europe.*

Kim, H. "Selecting the Optimal Gestational Carrier: Medical, Reproductive, and Ethical Considerations." *Fertility and Sterility* 113, no. 5 (2020): 892–96.

Klock, Susan C. "A Brief History of Donor Conception." *Psychology Today,* March 22, 2022.

Kostenzer, Julia, M. E. Bos, Annelies de Bont, and Jeroen van Exel. "Unveiling the Controversy on Egg Freezing in The Netherlands: A Q-Methodology Study on Women's Viewpoints." *Reproductive Biomedicine & Society Online* 12 (2020): 32–43.

Kramer, Wendy. "30k–60k US Sperm and Egg Donor Births Per Year?" *Huffington Post,* October 6, 2015; updated December 6, 2017.

"Las Donantes de Óvulos y Esperma: ¿Cuánto se Paga en Europa?" *Civio,* March 7, 2022.

Lee, Jessica C., Cheryl E. DeSantis, Stacey Boulet, and Jennifer F. Kawwass. "Embryo Donation: National Trends and Outcomes, 2004–2019." *American Journal of Obstetrics and Gynecology* 228, no. 3 (November 9, 2022): 318.e1–318.e7.

"Legislation about Egg Donation in Russia." *O.L.G.A. Fertility Clinic.*

Lowe, Sarah. "Marcia Cross Reveals She Tried a Sperm Donor." *Boston Herald,* February 14, 2008.

Luetkemeyer, L., and K. West. "Paternity Law: Sperm Donors, Surrogate Mothers, and Child Custody." *Missouri Medicine* 112, no. 3 (2015): 162–65.

McConnell, Julia. "Why Do Celebrities Use Surrogates: A Guide for Women and Couples." Family Creations (October 2, 2025).

Makler, Lauren. "Cofertility Donor Egg Options for Canadians." *Cofertility,* February 11, 2023; last modified May 21, 2025.

Mariwala, Trisha. "Anonymous Egg Donation Laws in the US and Abroad." *Cofertility,* December 19, 2022; last modified October 31, 2024.

Mariwala, Trisha. "Celebrities Who Have Used Donor Eggs." *Cofertility,* December 19, 2022; last modified October 31, 2024.

Nam, Chul Park. "Sperm Bank: From Laboratory to Patient." *World Journal of Men's Health* 36, no. 2 (2018): 89–91.

New York State Department of Health. "The Child-Parent Security Act: Gestational Surrogacy Agreements, Acknowledgment of Parentage and Orders of Parentage." *Vital Records,* revised February 2021.

O'Driscoll, Eliza. "What's Yours Is Mine." *The Guardian,* October 3, 2001.

Practice Committee of the American Society for Reproductive Medicine and Practice Committee for the Society for Assisted Reproductive Technology. "Gamete and Embryo Donation Guidance." *Fertility and Sterility* 111, no. 6 (2019): 1165–72.

Practice Committee of the American Society for Reproductive Medicine and Practice Committee of the Society for Assisted Reproductive Technology. "Recommendations for Practices Using Gestational Carriers: A Committee Opinion." *Fertility and Sterility* 118, no. 1 (2022): 65–74.

Practice Committee of the American Society for Reproductive Medicine and Practice Committee of the Society for Assisted Reproductive Technology. "Repetitive Oocyte Donation: A Committee Opinion." *Fertility and Sterility* 113, no. 6 (2020): 1150–53.

Preisler, L., N. Samara, Y. Kalma, and T. Arad. "Stringent Regulations of Oocyte Donation among Jewish Women in Israel: Characteristics and Outcomes of the National Oocyte Donation Program in One Central IVF Unit." *Journal of Religion and Health* 64, no. 1 (2024): 124–47.

"Purchasing and Consuming Tobacco." In "Mapping Minimum Age Requirements Concerning the Rights of the Child in the EU." *European Union Agency for Fundamental Rights*, November 20, 2017.

Rahim, Hannah. "Regulating International Commercial Surrogacy." *Petrie-Flom Center for Health Law Policy, Biotechnology, and Bioethics at Harvard Law School*, March 18, 2024.

Rajvanshi, Astha. "Why China Won't Allow Single Women to Freeze Their Eggs." *Time*, August 14, 2024.

"Reimbursing a Sperm or Ova (Egg) Donor or a Surrogate for Expenditures Related to Donation or Surrogacy." *Health Canada*, last modified June 9, 2020.

Rickman, Catherine. "Understanding the Drinking Age in France: Laws and Regulations." *Frenchly*, March 25, 2025.

"Rise of Egg and Sperm Donation Ends Heartache for Thousands, Says UK Regulator." *Human Fertilisation and Embryology Authority*, September 20, 2022.

Rodriguez, Bianca. "40 Celebrities Who Had Fertility Struggles." *Marie Claire*, July 22, 2021.

Rogalski, Jessica. "Sperm Donor Laws around the World." *Cryobank America*. December 1, 2023.

Santulli, Pietro, Paola Viganò, and Edgardo Somigliana. "Reimbursement of Elective Egg Freezing from Health Care Systems: Beyond Simplistic Claims." *International Journal of Gynecology & Obstetrics* 163, no. 1 (2023): 324–25.

Sarkar, Sonia. "Growing Numbers of Single Women in Islamic Countries Choosing to Freeze Eggs." *Religion Unplugged*, August 5, 2024.

"Selecting a Sperm Bank." *California Cryobank*.

Shvaikovsky, Maria. "Best Countries for Surrogacy in 2024: All You Need to Know" (blog). *International Fertility Group*, March 18, 2024.

Society for Assisted Reproductive Technology. *National Summary Report*. SART.

"Sperm Banking Background Fundamentals." *Fairfax Cryobank*.

"Sperm Banking History." *California Cryobank*.

"Sperm Donation and the Law." *NHS Sperm Donation*.

"Sperm Donation Laws by Country 2025." *World Population Review*.

"Surrogacy around the World." *Simple Surrogacy*, March 25, 2019.

"Surrogacy Laws by State." *Legal Professional Group of the American Society for Reproductive Medicine*, updated 2024.

Switzerland Tourism. "Alcohol and Tobacco." *MySwitzerland.com*.

VanHoose, Benjamin. "Actress Camille Guaty Reveals She's Pregnant After Using Egg Donor." *People*, June 23, 2021.

VanHoose, Benjamin. "Lance Bass Reveals Surrogate Suffered Miscarriage with Baby Boy at 8 Weeks." *People*, March 19, 2020.

"What You Need to Know about the History of Surrogacy." *American Surrogacy*.

"Which Countries Allow Commercial Surrogacy?" *Reuters*, April 5, 2023.

Wiecki, Aleksander. "Egg Donation in Spain: 2025 Costs, Availability & Clinics." *EggDonation Friends*, June 15, 2025.

"World Reports." *International Committee for Monitoring Assisted Reproductive Technologies (ICMART)*.

"Your Guide to How Many Eggs Can You Donate at a Time & How It Affects Your Overall Number of Eggs." *The World Egg and Sperm Bank*, January 18, 2023.

Chapter 7

"10 Sex Myths Busted by a Fertility Specialist." *Shady Grove Fertility*, January 23, 2023.

"Acupuncture and Infertility Treatment fact sheet." *American Society for Reproductive Medicine*, Patient Education Committee, 2015.

"Age and Fertility." *American Society for Reproductive Medicine*.

"Alcohol and Cancer Risk: The U.S. Surgeon General's Advisory." US Department of Health and Human Services, 2025.

Amable, Jody. "Fertility-Friendly Lubricants: What to Know and How to Choose." *Healthline*, August 18, 2025.

American Society for Reproductive Medicine. "Optimizing Natural Fertility: A Committee Opinion." *ASRM Practice Guidance*, December 2021.

American Society for Reproductive Medicine. "Performing the Embryo Transfer: A Guideline." *Fertility and Sterility* 107, no. 4 (2017): 882–96.

American Society for Reproductive Medicine. "Testing and Interpreting Measures of Ovarian Reserve: A Committee Opinion." *Fertility and Sterility* 114, no. 6 (December 2020): 1151–57.

Bentzen, Jens G., Jørgen L. Forman, Elisabeth C. Larsen, and Annette Pinborg. "Maternal Menopause as a Predictor of Anti-Müllerian Hormone Level and Antral Follicle Count in Daughters during Reproductive Age." *Human Reproduction* 28, no. 1 (2013): 247–55.

"Birth Control Pill FAQ: Benefits, Risks and Choices." *Mayo Clinic*, May 10, 2023.

"Bleeding during Pregnancy." *Cleveland Clinic*, August 27, 2024.

Coyle, Meaghan, Ieva Stupans, Khaled Abdel-Nour, et al. "Acupuncture versus Placebo Acupuncture for In Vitro Fertilisation: A Systematic Review and Meta-Analysis." *Acupuncture in Medicine* 39, no. 1 (2021): 20–29.

Cullinane, C., H. Gillan, J. Geraghty, et al. "Fertility Treatment and Breast-Cancer Incidence: Meta-Analysis." *BJS Open* 6, no. 1 (2022): zrab149.

Davis, Andrea R., Rachel Kroll, Beth Soltes, et al. "Occurrence of Menses or Pregnancy after

Cessation of a Continuous Oral Contraceptive." *Fertility and Sterility* 89, no. 5 (2008): 1059–63.

"Elective Egg Freezing." *CCRM Fertility.*

El-Toukhy, Tarek, S. K. Sunkara, M. Khairy, et al. "A Systematic Review and Meta-Analysis of Acupuncture in In Vitro Fertilisation." *BJOG: An International Journal of Obstetrics and Gynaecology* 115, no. 10 (2008): 1203–13.

Hovav, Karen. "Acupuncture for Improved Fertility: Is It Worth Trying?" *GoodRx Health*, July 27, 2022.

"Just the Facts: 'Restorative Reproductive Medicine' and 'Ethical IVF' Are Misleading Terms That Threaten Access." *American Society for Reproductive Medicine*, May 12, 2025.

Ku, Lowell. "Infertility in the Age of TikTok: Separating Fact from Fiction" (blog). *American Society for Reproductive Medicine (ASRM) News Tech Talk*, April 25, 2025.

Limiñana-Gras, Rosa M. "Health and Gender Perspective in Infertility." In *The Psychology of Gender and Health: Conceptual and Applied Global Concerns*, edited by M. Pilar Sánchez-López and Rosa M. Limiñana-Gras. Academic Press (Elsevier), 2017.

Lindberg, Sara. "Can These Self-Fertility Massages Help You Get Pregnant?" *Healthline*, April 22, 2020.

"Male Infertility: Causes, Symptoms, Tests & Treatment." *Cleveland Clinic*, January 25, 2024.

"Menopause: Symptoms and Causes." *Mayo Clinic.*

Melo, Patricia, Rupa Dhillon-Smith, Anjum Islam, et al. "Genetic Causes of Sporadic and Recurrent Miscarriage." *Fertility and Sterility* 120, no. 5 (2023): 940–44.

Nathan-Garner, Laura, and Kellie Bramlet. "The Pill and Cancer: Is There a Link?" *MD Anderson Cancer Center*, July 2016.

Novak, Sara. "Can a Fertility Massage Really Help You Get Pregnant?" *What To Expect,* February 25, 2022.

"Optimizing Natural Fertility." *American Society for Reproductive Medicine*, 2025.

"Optimizing Natural Fertility: Patient Education Fact Sheet." *American Society for Reproductive Medicine*, 2023.

"Ovarian Hyperstimulation Syndrome (OHSS): Causes & Treatment." *Cleveland Clinic*, December 5, 2023.

"Physical Activity and Exercise During Pregnancy and the Postpartum Period: Committee Opinion No. 804." *American College of Obstetricians and Gynecologists*, April 2020.

Practice Committee of the American Society for Reproductive Medicine. "Definition of Infertility: A Committee Opinion." *American Society for Reproductive Medicine*, 2023.

Practice Committee of the American Society for Reproductive Medicine. "Fertility Drugs and Cancer: A Guideline." *American Society for Reproductive Medicine*, 2024.

Practice Committee of the American Society for Reproductive Medicine. "Obesity and Reproduction: A Committee Opinion." *Fertility and Sterility* 116, no. 2 (2021): 377–84.

Practice Committee and Genetic Counseling Professional Group of the American Society for Reproductive Medicine. "Indications and Management of Preimplantation Genetic Testing for Monogenic Conditions: A Committee Opinion." *American Society for Reproductive Medicine*, 2023.

"Preconception Genetic Testing: Can It Assess Autism Risk?" *Orchid Health*, March 11, 2025.

Sapra, Kaitlyn J., Michael L. Eisenberg, Sungwoo Kim, et al. "Choice of Underwear and Male Fecundity in a Preconception Cohort of Couples." *Andrology* 4, no. 3 (2016): 500–8.

Smith, Caroline, Mike Armour, Zewdneh Shewamene, Hsiewe Ying Tan, Robert J. Norman, and Neil P. Johnson. "Acupuncture Performed around the Time of Embryo Transfer: A Systematic Review and Meta-Analysis." *Reproductive Biomedicine Online* 38, no. 3 (2019): 364–379.

Smith, Caroline, Sheryl de Lacey, Michael Chapman, et al. "Effect of Acupuncture vs Sham Acupuncture on Live Births among Women Undergoing In Vitro Fertilization." *JAMA* 319, no. 19 (2018): 1990–98.

"Tobacco or Marijuana Use and Infertility: A Committee Opinion." *American Society for Reproductive Medicine*, 2023.

Chapter 8

Domar, Alice, Kelly Smith, Catherine Conboy, et al. "A Prospective Investigation into the Reasons Why Insured United States Patients Drop Out of In Vitro Fertilization Treatment." *Fertility and Sterility* 94, no. 4 (2010): 1457–59.

Kreuzer, Verena K., Michael Kimmel, Jana Schiffner, et al. "Possible Reasons for Discontinuation of Therapy: An Analysis of 571,071 Treatment Cycles from the German IVF Registry." *Geburtshilfe und Frauenheilkunde* 78, no. 10 (2018): 984–90.

Kübler-Ross, Elisabeth. *On Death and Dying*. The MacMillan Company, 1969.

Rajkhowa, Manisha, Anne McConnell, and George E. Thomas. "Reasons for Discontinuation of IVF Treatment: A Questionnaire Study." *Human Reproduction* 21, no. 2 (2006): 358–63.

Van den Broeck, U., L. Holvoet, P. Enzlin, and E. Bakelants. "Reasons for Dropout in Infertility Treatment." *Gynecologic and Obstetric Investigation* 68, no. 1 (2009): 58–64.

Chapter 9

Bakalova, Daniela, Laura Navarro-Sanchez, and Carlos Rubio. "Non-Invasive Preimplantation Genetic Testing." *Genes* 16, no. 5 (2025): 552.

Chae-Kim, Jennifer, Nathan Doyle, Sahar Jahandideh, and John E. O'Brien. "Evaluating the Endometrial Receptivity Assay: A Nested Diagnostic Accuracy Study with the Synchrony Randomized Clinical Trial." *Fertility and Sterility* 120, no. 6 (2023): 1255–56.

Chavez-Badiola, Alejandro, Stephanie Kuku, and Joshua Abram. "The Potential of the Automated IVF Lab." *Fertility and Sterility*, July 10, 2025.

Fuller, Thomas. *A Pisgah-Sight of Palestine and the Confines Thereof*, 2nd ed. Printed by J. Flesher for J. Martyn and H. Herringman, 1650.

Grebe, Thomas A., Ghada Khusf, Jennifer M. Greally, et al. "Clinical Utility of Polygenic Risk Scores for Embryo Selection: A Points to Consider Statement of the American College of Medical Genetics and Genomics (ACMG)." *Genetics in Medicine* 26, no. 4 (2024): 101052.

Hajirasouliha, Iman, Josue Barnes, Nikica Zaninovic, Olivier Elemento, and Zev Rosenwaks. "Harnessing Artificial Intelligence Technology for IVF Embryo Selection." *Weill Cornell Medicine Newsroom*, December 19, 2022.

Kasaven, Laura, David Marcus, Eleni Theodorou, et al. "Systematic Review and Meta-Analysis: Does Pre-Implantation Genetic Testing for Aneuploidy at the Blastocyst Stage Improve Live Birth Rate?" *Journal of Assisted Reproduction and Genetics* 40, no. 10 (2023): 2297–316.

Mastenbroek, Sebastiaan, Moniek Twisk, Jannie van Echten-Arends, et al. "In Vitro Fertilization with Preimplantation Genetic Screening." *New England Journal of Medicine* 357, no. 1 (2007): 9–17.

National Academies of Sciences, Engineering, and Medicine; Health and Medicine Division; Board on Health Sciences Policy. *In Vitro–Derived Human Gametes as a Reproductive Technology: Scientific, Ethical, and Regulatory Implications: Proceedings of a Workshop*, edited by K. Bowman, C. Matney, and E. P. Dawson. National Academies Press, 2023.

Olawade, David B., Jennifer Teke, Khadijat K. Adeleye, Kusal Weerasinghe, Momudat Maidoki, and Aanuoluwapo Clement David-Olawade. "Artificial Intelligence in In-Vitro Fertilization (IVF): A New Era of Precision and Personalization in Fertility Treatments." *Journal of Gynecology Obstetrics and Human Reproduction* 54, no. 3 (2025): 102903.

Piechota, Sabrina, Maria Marchante, Alexa Giovannini, et al. "Human-Induced Pluripotent Stem Cell-Derived Ovarian Support Cell Co-Culture Improves Oocyte Maturation In Vitro after Abbreviated Gonadotropin Stimulation." *Human Reproduction* 38, no. 12 (2023): 2456–69.

Practice Committees of the American Society for Reproductive Medicine, the Society of Reproductive Biologists and Technologists, and the Society for Assisted Reproductive Technology. *In Vitro Maturation: A Committee Opinion. Fertility and Sterility* 115, no. 2 (2021): 298–304.

US Department of Labor, Wage and Hour Division. *Family and Medical Leave Act (FMLA)*.

Volovsky, Michael, Richard T. Scott, and Emre Seli. "Non-Invasive Preimplantation Genetic Testing for Aneuploidy: Is the Promise Real?" *Human Reproduction* 39, no. 9 (2024): 1898–1908.

Index